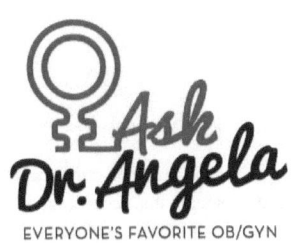

EVERYONE'S FAVORITE OB/GYN

WHAT TO EXPECT
During
PREGNANCY
and Beyond

ANGELA R. JONES, M.D.

Medical Disclaimer
All of the information provided throughout this book educating consumers about health and wellness are resources for educational and informational purposes only and should not take the place of consulting a physician. Purchase of this book does not create a doctor/patient relationship between the reader and Dr. Jones. This information is not intended to diagnose, treat, or cure a disease. This information does not and should not replace treatment from a medical professional.
If you need medical advice or assistance, you should consult a physician. If you are experiencing a medical emergency, DIAL 911. You should not act, or refrain from acting, on the basis of information included in this book without first consulting a licensed medical professional.

Ask. Dr. Angela: What to Expect During Pregnancy and Beyond
Angela R. Jones, MD

DEDICATION

First off, I'd like to thank God for His continued presence in my life. Two of my FAVE bible verses are: Greater is He that is in me, than he that is in the world. For I can do ALL things through Christ, who strengthens me. I thank Him for the desire. Will. Wherewithal to do what I do on a daily basis.

To my parents, who have and continue to lead by example. I thank you for the motivation. Support. Unwavering love. Sacrifice. Because of you, I am who I am, and am able to be the best mom I can be to my mini, Francesca. To my BEST girl in the whole world, my amazing daughter Francesca; none of this is possible without your unending love, support, sacrifice. Pregnancy was quite the experience for me, it changed my perspective on so many things ranging from pregnancy, motherhood, being an OB/GYN. Experience certainly is a good teacher. I am looking forward to our continued journey together as we travel along and deal with the numerous highs, lows, and surprises of life. Mom is the best title I have and it's all because of you.

To Hugh. Thank you for your continued belief in me and this project. Turns out I didn't need all the bells and whistles suggested by so many others. Just a continued belief in myself and this work. Looking forward to our next collaboration.

CONTENTS

Foreword by Lewis Weinstein, M.D.

Testimonials

Introduction

FOREWORD

Being a senior academic obstetrician gynecologist who is nearing the end of a potentially interesting career, one often wonders how much of an impact she/he may have had on others. This concept resulted in my most recent published editorial (American Journal of Obstetrics and Gynecology) called the 'Exponential Effect' about how the impact one has on another can spread far beyond what was expected. Nothing supports this concept more that the career of Angela Jones. I first met Angela while she was a medical student and I was Chairperson of the Department of Obstetrics & Gynecology at the University of Toledo College of Medicine. What caught my attention about Angela was her energy, enthusiasm, passion, caring nature and the fact that she had the biggest heart of any of her fellow students. Although medical school was a struggle for her, I was convinced that she would become an excellent physician.

We met numerous times during her school years and I was pleased that she decided to enter the field of obstetrics & gynecology. As one might write a Hollywood script, Angela had difficulty with passing structured examinations resulting in her not matching for a residency position. One of the few advantages of being a Chairperson (and there are not many) is the ability to make decisions that can markedly impact the future of another. Because of my ability to recognize a gemstone needing to be polished, I arranged for Angela to join our residency in Toledo. The rest is history, except for her continued difficulty with structured tests, but because of her profound drive, eventually all were successfully completed.

The result is an outstanding physician named Angela Jones who has been able to pass along to many others the knowledge and caring that was given to her. This is a classic example of the Exponential Effect and is what makes an old person feel that all their efforts were of some benefit and brings a smile to an old wrinkled face.

After reading this book by Angela "*What to Expect During Pregnancy and Beyond*", I truly understood what the word 'practical' means. The definition of practical is "of or concerned with the actual doing or use of something rather than with theory and ideas." This book written in a clear humorous manner gives the reader all the correct answers as what to expect during her pregnancy. The practicality is superb, and humor made me laugh numerous times and blurt out to myself, "boy is that Angela."

This is the type of book that should become a bible to all pregnant patients irrespective of their educational level. The information presented is clear, concise and most important, ACCURATE. I advise any woman contemplating pregnancy to read this book. You will laugh many times but come away far more knowledgeable after the read and better able to understand the profound changes that your body will undergo during the miraculous process of giving life to another human being.

When I finished reading the book, I was ecstatic that the decision that I made to give Angela the opportunity that she so richly deserved had worked out far beyond my expectations. Read the book; laugh and learn. Then I can also add you to my collection of those affected by the Exponential Effect.

Louis Weinstein, MD

Past Bowers Professor and Chair, Department of Obstetrics & Gynecology

Thomas Jefferson University

Philadelphia, PA

TESTIMONIALS

Dr. Angela is the best doctor I've ever had. She is wonderful with patient interaction, makes you feel comfortable to ask any questions you may have and answers them with very thoughtful responses. I was lucky to have her as part of my care for post-delivery care in the hospital and after. She always is funny and makes you laugh and relax during your appointments.
Kelly Aaron Mager

So happy to have had Dr. Jones deliver my baby girl a few weeks ago! She is kind hearted, extremely knowledgeable, and was a big cheerleader during delivery. After all that, during appointments she makes you so comfortable you feel like you are talking to your girlfriends. Great doctor!!
Katie Matecki Maits

No one compares! Most professional kindest person in health care! Love this lady.
Crystal Marie

Dr. Angela was understanding and supportive of my choices during my pregnancy, and when it didn't happen as I'd hoped, she was there for me then, too. Easy to talk to and extremely patient, I've never had a doctor like her!
Susan Reistrom

The most approachable doctor I've ever met. Thank you and keep up the good work. The world needs more doctors like you.
Chi Arguelles

INTRODUCTION

"It was all a dream - I used to read Word Up! magazine..."

That's the Notorious B.I.G. aka Biggie Smalls -- baby, baby, I love that song! All right, confession: I love anything to do with babies! I'll always find a way to make even the mere mention of babies fit into my world, even if it is an out of context classic '90s hip-hop classic.

All jokes aside, my life really is a dream. Not just mine, but my aunts', uncles', parents', grandparents', and great-grandparents' who did not have anywhere near the opportunities that I have been afforded.

I'm here because of them.

I'm Dr. Angela, a tiny, woman of color (I'm not sure what the politically correct terminology is anymore; I suppose it depends on who you're speaking with, you know, some of us can get away with saying certain things) with a HUGE voice. No, really, just ask my daughter who is constantly reminding me to use my "inside" voice, when, truth be told, my inside voice just happens to be incredibly loud. Don't believe me? Then ask the long list of assistants and nurses I've worked with who already have the scripts, orders, and instructions ready for patients before they ever leave my rooms. I guess my inside voice can't be contained in four walls. It's just that I get so very excited about whatever it is I'm trying to convey.

I was born to be Dr. Angela!

From the age of four I knew, and professed to whomever would listen, that I wanted to be a physician. I was born and primarily raised in Columbus, Ohio by my mom. She did all the things she was supposed to do, she kept me clothed, fed, a roof over my head, and most of all, loved. Even before all the fancy degrees and unlimited resources, I learned that faith, love, and prayer were enough to get me by.

When I was sixteen, I decided to move to Cincinnati to live with my father and other mom. (I don't believe in terms such as "step-mom." My father's second wife has always treated me and loved me as if I was her own) Even at this young age I knew that a move to Cincinnati was necessary for me to achieve my goal of becoming a physician. My dad always promised me that he would do everything in his power to help me reach that goal, and he and my mom sacrificed to make sure I received the best education possible. I remember my dad wore the same pair of dress shoes for, like, four years. He just had them resoled. Private schools can be expensive, and when you work for the Lord as a pastor, like my father, the reward is not in this lifetime, but the next. I remember the embarrassment I used to feel when he dropped me off at school in the church van. It became a running joke, I remember my friends yelling, "Ang, your dad's here," as the Jesus mobile parallel parked up the block.

But pride for my family outweighed any kind of silly teenage shame. My pops was there. He has always been there, through every stage of my life.

I remember not being sure where I would go to undergrad. I had applied for and won a partial scholarship to Boston University and had been accepted into their college of engineering (I have always had a love of math and science). The thought was that I would get a degree in biomedical engineering and then go to medical school. Nevertheless, even with the scholarship it was still too expensive. I remember one day in late August 1990, still unsure where I would attend college, my dad encouraged me to interview at a small, liberal arts school in Danville, Kentucky. I was so pissed! Why would I, a black woman, want to go to school in some rinky-dink Kentucky town where I would, once again, be one of only a handful of black folk? I interviewed in a tie-dyed t-shirt and cut up jeans, but amazingly, Centre College gave me a full academic scholarship. I played three years of varsity field hockey (I had never played the sport in my life but saw it on a brochure in the president of the university's office and thought it might be fun) and became one of the 90-something percent of their graduates with pre-med majors that went on to medical school. I was honored to be chosen by my graduating class to speak on their behalf at our convocation.

Medical school and residency, though they offered periods of fun, were complete ass kickers. Most people have no idea the amount of sacrifice involved in getting a medical degree. There are entire chapters in the history of my family that I missed because I was hard at work studying. There are times when I go home and look at family photos that I'm not in. It's funny when on-lookers see the pictures and don't realize there is someone missing: me. My family has to remind them, "We have another daughter."

Well, I'm not missing anymore! I have arrived, so to speak. This job demands a lot, and even though the sacrifices made by myself and my family are indescribable at best---long hours in the office, being on-call, weekends and holidays spent away---my work is, undeniably, a labor of love. There's no other reason I would do it.

It's funny how things come full circle. Once upon a time I wrote in a medical school essay that I wanted to be the editor-in chief of a women's magazine that was to have the auspicious name Annie Rae (my dear friend Dr. Gina Jefferson calls me that to this day). Lo and behold, it has manifested. Not as Annie Rae, but as the Ask Dr. Angela Podcast on iTunes, the Ask Dr. Angela blog, the Ask Dr. Angela website, and now a book by me, Dr. Angela.

I LOVE TO WRITE! Whether it's scribbling in my journal or having my poetry published for greeting cards (Blue Mountain Arts, y'all), the written word has always been a formidable means of expression for me. You know, sometimes you've just got to GET IT OUT! I have a lot to get out. Did I also mention that I have a lot to say?

That and I LOVE WOMEN! Now, this may seem obvious, me having a wife and all, but really, being a woman is some impressive s&*t! I continue to be amazed, on a regular basis, by the beauty of women, the strength of women, the drive, grace, and perseverance that is involved with being a woman. I bear witness on a daily basis as to why God made a woman who and what she is. AMAZING! We are built to take a licking and keep on ticking.

You indescribably strong women, I wrote this book for you! Pregnancy is already stressful enough, so I want to provide a resource that is light, fun, easy to read, and even easier to understand. Over the course of several years I have compiled a list of the most common questions I address while seeing women for their prenatal visits. I've seen the books my patients rely on for insight and answers throughout this journey called pregnancy. I have personally found them to be intimidating, long, cumbersome, and, most importantly, boring! Talk about a snooze fest! I also think that most of those books provide way more information than the average woman needs to know. Sometimes knowing too much is not a good thing (you're not the only one who has self-diagnosed a bug bite as a cancerous tumor thanks to aggressive web searching).

This book is my way of letting you know that we're in this thing together, not only because I am a doctor, but because I am a mother, too, and I know what you're going through.

I remember the long drives back and forth between Toledo, Ohio and our doctor's office in Michigan. It was a nearly 45-minute trek. I remember the day that we were inseminated with my mini-me. We knew that things had "taken" immediately when I started feeling nauseated right off the bat. I remember peeing on that stick and seeing a smiley face. We were pregnant! I remember driving back and forth to Michigan for blood work (boy, did I hate all that hormone level testing) and ultrasounds. I remember the first day we saw that heartbeat on the ultrasound. We were (and still are) overjoyed. We know it all. Documented it all. Everything from when I felt my first wave of nausea to when we first saw the peanut on the ultrasound screen to when we first felt her move, to determining when she would be born.

My wife and I always tell our little girl that there isn't much we don't know about her. In fact, we have her down to a T because we documented everything that happened while she was growing inside me. Everything from the way she sighs and abruptly turns away when she's annoyed to how her personality goes right out the window when she's tired or hungry seems to be something we knew about her before she even came to be. We planned for little Miss Francesca, who is every bit a Francesca and not the Frankie that we thought we'd be calling her.

I've been there. I get it.

Whether it be funny stories, anecdotes, and experiences from my own pregnancy, or hardcore medical information, you will get it all.

As a mother, wife, and OB/GYN, I see, hear, and experience some enlightening, hilarious, and outrageous things. I'm sure you know the feeling, girl. Welcome to my world! And thank you for letting me into yours.

I hope you enjoy reading this as much as I enjoyed writing it!

Now off to strum my guitar.

Dr. Angela.

CHAPTER 1
HEALTH AND BEAUTY

Drinking during pregnancy

I had the privilege of meeting a pregnant woman the other day (imagine that). She was in her second trimester of pregnancy. On this particular occasion, the woman asked, "Dr. Angela, do you think it would be okay if I had a drink?" My immediate response was, "A drink of what?" She then beckoned me over with her hand and whispered in my ear, "I've been dying for a glass of red wine!"

I know that some of you are likely thinking, "Alcohol during pregnancy, that's a no brainer." Well, not so much! Many folks seem to be under the impression that a sip here or a glass of wine there will have no impact on the unborn fetus.

WRONG! I DO NOT, under any circumstances, recommend that my pregnant moms knowingly consume alcohol, regardless of what trimester they are in! The American Academy of Pediatrics recently released data implicating fetal alcohol exposure as the leading PREVENTABLE cause of birth defects and intellectual/neurodevelopmental problems in children.

How much alcohol does it take to cause such issues? No one knows for sure, so it's best to just avoid alcohol altogether. Here's what you need to know about Fetal Alcohol Spectrum Disorder, formerly known as Fetal Alcohol Syndrome:

IT'S PREVENTABLE! Just say no to alcohol during pregnancy!

Fetal Alcohol Spectrum Disorder shows up as a combination of mental, physical, and behavioral problems. It may cause physical abnormalities including, but not limited to, small head, a smooth philtrum (the space between the nose and the upper lip) and shorter than normal height. In addition, neurodevelopmental effects such as low IQ, behavioral issues, and attention deficit disorders are common.

Structural and/or functional disorders with organ systems such as the heart, kidneys, and bones are also commonplace in this disorder. Hearing and

1

vision may also be affected. The more you drink, the more likely you are to have a child with Fetal Alcohol Spectrum Disorder.

Newsflash: LEGAL AND SAFE DON'T NECESSARILY GO HAND IN HAND!

Comparatively speaking, alcohol produces more significant neurobehavioral effects in the fetus than drugs such as heroin, cocaine, or marijuana. Twenty percent of pregnant women consume alcohol, and often where there is the use of one substance, there are likely to be others.

So, don't get your panties in a bunch when I inquire about the use of alcohol or drugs as if it couldn't be you -- it could be ANYONE! I'm just saying, don't let it be you.

Can I dye my hair during pregnancy?

HELL TO THE YEAH! I love this question. While you will often hear me mention pregnancy being amazingly wonderful and all that good stuff, the toll it takes on your body isn't quite that. That's not to say that pregnancy is miserable for all parties involved, it's just that during my pregnancy I seemed to have every ache, pain, sleepless night, craving, and heartburn imaginable. Having said such, with everything that an expectant mother goes through, it's very important that she feel good about herself. My wife and I always refer to "face, body, and fashion," specifically referring to women that have it together. One of the reasons I forego the traditional white, starched doctor's coat in the office and dress to impress is that it makes me feel so much better. Makeup and hair are a big part of that. I didn't dye my hair during pregnancy because I just didn't have the time, however, it's okay to do so if you so desire. I totally get roots growing out, highlights looking jacked up, and just feeling crazy about your mane. If you are one of those people who are super concerned about the potential side effects of dyeing your hair during pregnancy, just wait until the second trimester, that way most of the important development has occurred with regard to organogenesis. There is NO HARD DATA suggesting that hair dyes, or the chemicals in them, pose any threat to a developing fetus.

You could also consider doing things like streaking (I guess this has made a comeback), highlighting, frosting (shout out to the original Charlie's Angels), or other techniques where the dye doesn't come into direct contact with the scalp. If you are a DIY kinda gal, make sure that you observe the obvious precautions like rinsing the color out of your hair when recommended, wearing gloves, and making certain that you are in a well-ventilated area.

Is one prenatal vitamin better than the others?

Though I'm sure there are many drug companies that would love me to plug their particular formulations, I can't honestly say that there is any one prenatal vitamin that is better than another. The prenatal vitamin that is best for you is going to be the one that you can swallow with ease (have you seen prenatal vitamins? Some of them are like horse pills), and doesn't make you nauseated, gassy, constipated, or sick. If swallowing pills isn't your thing, there are chewable options. Affordability will also be a factor as prenatal vitamins can be expensive.

Quite frankly, I've had moms that ended up taking Flintstone vitamins as a result of not being able to tolerate traditional prenatal vitamins. While I am by no means advocating Barney Rubble as pregnancy guru, I say it to say this: There is no best prenatal vitamin. Just ensure that what you do take has the adequate amount of folic acid in it, 400 mcg, and that, if possible, you initiate it before you even become pregnant! I always encourage my ladies to begin taking prenatal vitamins when they stop taking birth control. That way your body already has everything onboard to ensure that baby has what it needs in the early, most critical, stages of development.

What meds can I take during pregnancy?

All too often I see the long-suffering expectant mother playing the role of martyr and enduring common ailments such as headaches, heartburn, cold, flu, constipation, and back pain. She may be afraid of medications having harmful effects on her developing fetus. The struggle is real but the good news is there's no need to endure it! If you choose not to take any medications because that's just you, then so be it. But for those of you who just aren't sure what to do and what is or isn't safe, I'll tell you like I tell my patients, YOU BETTER ASK SOMEBODY! Pregnancy, however smooth, is going to be a wild ride, but there are some things we can do to help make it a bit more tolerable. Let's start with:

Headaches: If you have a history of migraines, pregnancy may affect them a number of different ways. They may get better, worse, or remain about the same. Be sure to check with your physician to confirm what meds are safe to take as a number of medications used to treat migraines are not recommended for use in the pregnant state. I recommend Tylenol (you can even take extra strength) as directed. If regular ol' Tylenol doesn't do the trick, you might consider chasing it with your favorite caffeinated drink (Mountain Dew, Coke, coffee). If those offer no relief, a visit with your OB/GYN might be in order as there are certain medical conditions (preeclampsia comes to mind), where persistent headaches may be a sign. We also may need to consult our friendly neurologist to see if we can't better control your migraine, if indeed that is the issue.

Allergies: Don't you just hate seasonal allergies? I know I do. Honestly, never had them prior to moving to New Jersey. As if gas, heartburn and swelling, weren't enough, now the stuffy nose, runny eyes, and cough. ARE YOU KIDDING ME? Try some Benadryl, Claritin, or Zyrtec. Saline nasal spray may also be helpful.

Back Pain: Let me just start by saying it gets worse before it gets better. Needless to say, I get a lot of side eye glances and "screw you" huffs with the aforementioned statement. Don't kill the clinical messenger! Stress on the lower back is very common in pregnancy due to the shift in your center of gravity. As the uterus continues to grow and show, there is an obvious stress and exaggeration of the curvature in your lower back. There is also an increase in sciatic nerve aggravation, again, caused by this gradual shift in your center of gravity. With all those joints, bones, and ligaments becoming much more lax as a result of the hormones of pregnancy, no wonder you may be experiencing some nerve compression, which usually translates into radiating pain down one leg. What to do? Some of my common recommendations include using a pillow for lower back support while driving or sitting at your desk or dinner table. A maternity belt for uterine support may help to support your growing uterus, which in turn will take some of the stress off your lower back. Warm compresses and heating pads (not too hot!) to the lower back not only feel great but may also provide some relief. In addition, let's not forget about a good old-fashioned massage! This may be a good time to get the partners involved. Most of our partners may feel pretty useless up to this point as they have NO IDEA of all the discomfort you're currently enduring, so put them to good use and order up some back massages. This is also a circumstance where I can refer to my friendly chiropractors. I have a few friends that are chiropractors and they take excellent care of my pregnant ladies. Not to fear, they are not going to manipulate you into labor. They have proven to be a valued resource in my battle against back pain in pregnancy.

Swelling: THIS IS NO LONGER A PART OF THE DIAGNOSTIC CRITERIA FOR PREECLAMPSIA! Once upon a time it was, but not anymore. All pregnant moms get swelling in their extremities. As long as one extremity isn't more swollen than the other, and there is no associated pain (these could be signs of a clot), there's not too much to worry about. Propping your feet up when you have an opportunity can also relieve swelling. Support hose are helpful, though at times they can be incredibly annoying, especially if it's hot outside. Then again, I feel that way wearing them even when I'm not pregnant.

Cold/Flu: First off, I recommend that ALL my pregnant moms get the flu shot. Second, most of what you do for a cold when you're pregnant is what you did for a cold when you weren't. Pregnancy brain be damned, we will remember all the stuff our mothers used to tell us. So, fluids, fluids, and more fluids. I like Gatorade (the blue and purple are my personal favorites), water, Pedialyte (I have never been able to tolerate the taste of Pedialyte, but if you're throwing your brains up, it's a good way to help replace electrolytes), ginger ale, or 7Up. You know, OLD-SCHOOL. Tylenol (extra strength if needed) is good for aches and pains, saline nasal spray for dry nasal passages, a humidifier to stave off dry air, Robitussin (DM if needed), and Mucinex are a few of the meds I have in my arsenal. I don't tend to recommend meds that contain pseudoephedrine/phenylephrine. These are contained in certain decongestants like Sudafed. Remember, if these conservative measures don't work or you feel as if your symptoms are getting worse, contact your OB/GYN.

Nausea/Vomiting: To combat this I recommend small, frequent meals and a pretty boring diet at best. Have you ever heard of the BRAT diet? That's bananas, rice, applesauce, and toast. Start with these things and advance your diet as needed. I would avoid spicy foods and eats that are high in acidity. Ginger is great for nausea -- ginger ale, ginger snaps, or even ginger candies. As far as medications are concerned, the only FDA approved medication currently on the market for nausea is Diclegis. Zofran is no longer in my arsenal due to its association with cleft palates and cardiac defects. Reglan is another medication that I commonly prescribe for nausea during pregnancy. It's usually taken 30 minutes before meals and at bedtime. As always, if none of the above are working or you feel as if things are getting worse, contact your OB/GYN.

Constipation: TOTALLY SUCKS! The hormones of pregnancy wreak havoc on all systems of your body. Not only does the slowing of the digestive tract lead to things like heartburn and delayed emptying of the gallbladder, which can lead to a sludge and/or stone formation (um, can we say ouch), but it can also lead to constipation! The deal with constipation is that if your bowels aren't regular it's usually the cause of lower abdominal pain and cramping. Whenever I have a pregnant mom complaining of lower abdominal cramping I always inquire about bowel function. As previously stated, the hormones of pregnancy tend to slow things down. To help keep things moving I encourage diets that are high in fiber, lots of fruits and vegetables, as well as fiber supplementation. My over-the-counter recommendations are Colace and, my personal favorite, Citrucel (get the citrus flavor).

Diarrhea: If it's not coming out of one end, it's the other, amiright?! While you may have GI (gastrointestinal) bugs that will eventually run their 24-hour course, it's important to remain hydrated. Dehydration can lead to an unhappy uterus that often translates into cramping or contractions. The previously mentioned BRAT diet is good for diarrhea and trying to bulk up stools. You may also consider Imodium. If your symptoms don't resolve or improve within a 24-hour period, it's important to follow up with your OB/GYN.

Carpal Tunnel Syndrome: At some point during your pregnancy you may or may not start feeling, and this is a direct quote, "LIKE A f&%#in' WHALE!" Especially with all the swelling in your legs, feet, hands, and fingers. Are you still wearing your rings? It's not uncommon to feel numbness/tingling/pain in your hands and/or wrists, especially at night. Carpal tunnel syndrome is a common occurrence during pregnancy, mostly during the second half. With all the extra fluid and swelling associated with pregnancy, the symptoms commonly associated with this syndrome are due to nerve compression. Most of what we recommend for relief is pretty conservative. Perhaps wearing a splint at night, avoiding activities that might aggravate it, like typing, and, in especially severe cases, steroid injections.

Gas: Gotta love pregnancy. As beautiful as pregnancy is, it is not the most comfortable state of being. Talk about being a lady going right out the door. I never burped and farted so much in my lifetime! While I pride myself on being every bit of a lady---you know, always paying attention to "carriage;" whether in a skirt, dress, or heels, a lady always has to carry herself a certain way---needless to say, a lot of that was pretty much null and void during pregnancy! Paying close attention to your diet and avoiding foods associated with gas, like beans, carbonated drinks, dairy products, and fatty snacks, will help. Eating too fast and chewing gum are activities associated with gas production, so slow down. Avoiding them will prove to be beneficial. And while being mindful of all this good stuff may help, medicinal options I commonly recommend include over the counter remedies like Gas-X and Tums.

Insomnia: I typically encounter two different sleeping scenarios with the pregnancies I see. One is during the first half of the pregnancy when expectant moms aren't sleeping because they are afraid of hurting the baby. "OMG, I woke up and was sleeping on my stomach," or "OMG, I woke up lying flat on my back," or "OMG, I was sleeping on my right side."

The second, surprisingly enough, occurs during the second half of pregnancy and is about not being able to get comfortable, or just not being able to fall asleep. Let's deal with the first scenario.

I typically tell my moms-to-be TO JUST SLEEP! Trust that your body will tell you how to lay. At some point, you will no longer be able to comfortably sleep on your stomach or your back due to the changes your body is undergoing, such as your growing uterus, and the increasing curvature of your lower back (remember we spoke of this a few sections back when discussing back pain?). Until then, as long as you aren't making any conscious efforts to lie flat on your stomach or back, JUST SLEEP! If you happen to wake up on your right side, on your back, or on your stomach during the early part of your pregnancy, DON'T FREAK OUT. Remember, baby isn't just under your skin, there's skin, subcutaneous fat, fascia, muscle, peritoneum, uterus, amniotic sac, and then baby! Lots and lots of protective layers.

Regarding the second scenario, and I've said this a million times, you know, about pregnancy not being the most comfortable state of being, I recommend body pillows that conform to your body and all the crazy positions I'm sure you're trying in your efforts to get cozy. If this fails, Benadryl is a good option (am I the only one that had a mom or knew grown folks that used to slip their children Benadryl to "calm them down?"). Though I don't often recommend it, Unisom is also an option.

Itching: HYDRATE, HYDRATE, HYDRATE! Remember, the skin is your body's largest organ; staying well hydrated will certainly help with this.

There is no need to invest in all those fancy schmancy lotions, potions, and elixirs. Using a heavy cream or lotion will usually do the trick. Aveeno is good, but my personal favorites are simple, natural cocoa and shea butters. They're easy to apply and easy on the wallet.

Another trick that I love is using baby oil prior to drying off. I recommend rinsing off in the shower, and while your skin is still moist, covering your entire body with baby oil. Be careful, now, it can get slippery. After the initial application, pat yourself dry with your washcloth. My skin was so soft and smooth using this little at-home spa treatment. I didn't even get any stretch marks!

If none of the above works and you are still itching, you may want to let your OB/GYN know as there are some serious diagnoses, such as Cholestasis of pregnancy, which can be associated with itching.

What foods can I eat and what foods should I avoid during pregnancy?

I am such a foodie it's crazy. I'm always asking my pregnant moms what's on the menu for the night or what was served for breakfast (hungry gynos want to know!). I've certainly gotten a dinner idea or two from my expectant moms when I've blanked out on ideas (shh, don't tell my wife). I've also gotten some great tips on restaurants and local joints that are off the beaten path. Between my love affair with good eats and all the cravings and aversions that come with any normal pregnancy, my own diet while I was carrying consisted of lots of breakfast foods (I couldn't get enough of turkey bacon, French toast, waffles, eggs) and, well, I'm really embarrassed to share this, but I consumed so many DQ Blizzards and 7/11 Slurpees that I should've bought stock. On a more serious note, in pregnancy I have found that it's not so much about what you can eat, but more about what foods to avoid. My take home for expectant moms is to focus on eating a well-balanced, healthy, diet. Healthy translates differently for everyone. As long as your diet considers the following, you should be good to go:

Tuna: Just say no! I've always told my pregnant moms to avoid tuna, fresh and canned, as there have always been questions about mercury content. While there continues to be a debate on whether tuna is or isn't one of the low mercury choices, other yummy, safe seafood options you can eat during pregnancy are salmon, tilapia, shrimp, and sardines. Remember, seafood is an excellent source of lean protein as well as essential fatty acids that are necessary for the neurological development of the growing fetus. Hence, the recommendation isn't to avoid fish altogether, just to make informed choices.

Eggs and Meat: Everything you consume needs to be WELL DONE! Nothing raw or undercooked. No runny eggs or rare meats. If you consume lunchmeat, it must be cooked! Either go panini-style, nuke it in the microwave, fry it, or grill it. It doesn't matter how it's cooked, IT JUST NEEDS TO BE PIPING HOT and not straight out of the refrigerator or deli. The concern here is for listeria, which can have some pretty serious consequences for both mother and baby during pregnancy.

Cow's Milk: All dairy and milk products must be pasteurized! Soft cheeses such as brie, feta, and bleu cheese, unless clearly labeled as pasteurized, should be avoided.

PS: Avoid drinking unpasteurized juices!

The above are pretty straightforward and easy to follow for most; unless you are a frequent shopper at the farmer's market or someone who buys things from folks selling goods straight off the farm or on the side of the road.

Should I stop taking my antidepressant medications now that I'm pregnant?

Great question, which leads me to first plug the importance of preconception counseling.

Prior to getting pregnant, I ideally like to meet with my moms-to-be to review medical history, medications, family, and social history. All this to ensure you are in your best possible state to endure and enjoy a safe pregnancy. This intake may include getting rid of habits placing you at an increased risk, such as being overweight or smoking. Thoroughly reviewing medications to ensure their safety and perhaps finding alternatives to those not deemed safe during pregnancy also occurs at preconception counseling visits.

Having said such, I do NOT recommend pregnant moms stopping their meds cold turkey without first consulting a physician. First of all, it might pose a risk to you, secondly, not treating a medical condition that needs to be treated might have an adverse effect on both you and baby. Depression is a great example of this. If left untreated, depression can have a significant impact on a pregnancy, whether it's a mom not showing up for prenatal visits, not eating, or not sleeping. Do the math. You can see how such behavior would and could impact a pregnancy. The point I'm trying to make is this: When taking medications during pregnancy, the pros and cons are always weighed. While there are certain medications that are safer than others, your physician should be an integral part of the decision to continue or discontinue your medications.

What can I use to clean my face during pregnancy?

Are you familiar with that old wives' tale about boys protecting their mothers' beauty while in utero? So it says, women give off that "pregnancy glow" because male fetuses want their mothers to be beautiful, whereas girls steal their mother's beauty. Hence, the terrible acne and enhanced symptoms of pregnancy that so many women experience with having a daughter. Well, words were never truer than in the case of my own pregnancy. My daughter totally KICKED MY BUTT! I had the worst skin ever. You wanna talk about acne? This was on a completely different level! Plus, I had every ache and pain imaginable. My little one certainly took everything I had because she turned out to be absolutely gorgeous.

The hormones of pregnancy wreak havoc on so many different levels. I mean, the obvious things are the breast pain, mood and emotional labilities, back pain, and heartburn, but let's not forget about the acne that so often plagues so many during pregnancy. I hated it! When it comes to skin care during pregnancy, less is more. Keep it simple. You don't need any of those overpriced skin care systems. A gentle cleanser used twice daily, along with an oil-free moisturizer, will usually suffice.

I loved the Aveeno products when I was pregnant. I recommend that you use your hands to wash your face instead of a washcloth to avoid irritating or aggravating the skin. Make sure that you thoroughly rinse and pat your skin dry. I was and still am a huge fan of witch hazel pads. They're sort of old-school, I know, but for those of you that know me, you know that I love to mix the old with the new. I think the witch hazel pads are a nice way to cleanse the skin of any "extra" oils and dirt. Bonus, it makes skin feel cool and soothed, and completely cleared my skin of my pregnancy acne.

Being mindful of your diet, avoiding fatty and fried foods, sugars, and consuming plenty of water will also help you maintain radiant skin during the course of your pregnancy.

Anything containing isotretinoin should be avoided during pregnancy. Also, try to avoid popping pimples. As annoying as they are, you'll be sorry if you pop them, leaving behind scars as unpleasant reminders. If your acne is so bad that you just can't bear the sight of it, you might consider seeing a dermatologist to learn about certain antibiotics that are safe to use during pregnancy.

Can I exercise during pregnancy?

HELL YEAH! Please excuse my brashness. You all know my catch phrase, "Is baby movin' and groovin'?" Well how about is baby's momma movin' and groovin'? Exercise during pregnancy really DOES THE BODY AND PREGNANCY GOOD! I know, I know, you're tired all the time, your back hurts, your legs are swollen, the list goes on and on and on, but guess what? Exercising will help you feel so much better. Exercise will actually give you more energy, stamina, and help you to sleep better at night.

So, now you're asking the million-dollar question, WHAT TYPES OF EXERCISES CAN I DO DURING PREGNANCY? Lucky for you expectant ladies, there are plenty of exercises that you can do during pregnancy. Walking is always a good one, then there's prenatal yoga or treadmill work. Non-weight-bearing exercises such as the elliptical machine and stationary bike are also smart choices. Swimming is great for moms-to-be, as it doesn't place a lot of stress on your bones, joints or ligaments. Even weight training, to a degree, as long as you don't overdo it -- please, no 200-lb. deadlifting. I recommend avoiding any activities or exercises that require a lot of balance and thus increase your risk of falling. I would also stay away from any exercises that require you to lie flat on your back after 20 weeks gestation (goodbye sit-ups, hello baby).

Try to exercise at least 30 minutes daily and make sure you are drinking plenty of fluids along the way. If you start feeling tired, dizzy, or lightheaded, either stop or lessen the intensity of your workout.

As in the non-pregnant state, exercise is a lifestyle modifying activity. I can't begin to emphasize the importance of exercise. I once heard someone say "EXERCISE IS MEDICINE!" It is preventative at best! Exercising will help curb weight gain and the likelihood of developing things like gestational diabetes, high blood pressure in pregnancy, and postpartum depression.

Word to the wise: If you have any pre-existing medical diagnoses or pregnancy issues that might be adversely impacted by exercise, please check with your OB/GYN prior to beginning your exercise program.

Is bleeding normal after intercourse?
Is it safe to have sex during pregnancy?

First off, let's address the obvious. Sex is fine during pregnancy, granted you haven't been placed on pelvic rest and you and your partner can get over the mental aspect of it -- fear of hurting the baby! I find that lots of husbands, guy friends, partners, spouses in general, have some subconscious fear of hurting their baby during sex. Trust me buddy, you won't come anywhere close to hitting the baby, if you know what I mean.

Pregnancy sex can be some of the best you've ever had. You might even find that you want it more! Sex while pregnant will challenge you to be creative, as you'll be working around a growing uterus. Twister anyone?

As previously mentioned, everything is super vascular during pregnancy, your cervix included, so you may notice a small amount of spotting post-intercourse. This typically isn't anything to write home about as long as there is no active bleeding, which could signal certain things such as an infection or issue with placental location. If you notice active bleeding, you should call/see your OB/GYN pronto!

Can I still get my nails/toes done during pregnancy?

A resounding YES! After all, a girl's still gotta be a girl! Just be safe about it. By that I mean, go to salons that are well-ventilated and practice good hygiene. You know what I'm talking about: thoroughly cleansing the foot bowls and hand soaks in between uses, good sterilization techniques regarding instruments and tools. Lots of women get acrylics, and while there is no hard evidence suggesting that they or the chemicals used to apply them are harmful to the developing fetus, why not take advantage of those pregnancy hormones, which should be making your nails grow naturally long and strong.

If the salon isn't quite your thing, try having your significant other give you an at-home mani/pedi. Those toes get awfully difficult to reach once you're in the third trimester.

Total aside, but as an OB/GYN I enjoy seeing pretty hands and feet.

What can I do to prevent stretch marks during my pregnancy?

Stretch marks! I can't tell you how many home remedies, creams, lotions, potions, and elixirs I've seen or heard of, all claiming to prevent stretch marks. These human tiger stripes occur when the body grows at a rate faster than its skin can keep up with. Pregnancy is a prime example of rapid cell growth and turnover.

Hydrate. Hydrate. Hydrate. The skin is our largest organ! Ensuring that your skin is hydrated enough to help with the constant sloughing off of dead cells and regeneration of the new goes a long way. Remember, it's easier to stretch something that is soft and elastic as opposed to dry and brittle. HYDRATE!

Moisturize. Moisturize. Moisturize. Did I say MOISTURIZE? Heavy lotions, creams, butters (shea or cocoa), or oils will suffice. Anything that makes your skin feel soft, smooth, and less itchy will do the trick. Don't get caught up spending a fortune on products that claim miracles.

And of course, maintain a healthy diet. You really are what you eat.

Weight gain during pregnancy -- how much is enough?

The amount of weight that you should gain during pregnancy is actually determined by your pre-pregnancy body mass index (BMI). In case you're scratching your head and wondering what the heck that is, your BMI is calculated by dividing your weight in kilograms by your height in meters squared. BMI = $kg/m2$. Because wellness and overall fitness is an important piece of what's discussed at most of my visits, pregnant or not, if you've seen me, this is likely familiar to you.

BMI < 18.5 is considered to be underweight; recommended weight gain is 28 to 40 pounds

BMI 18.5 - 24.9 is considered normal; recommended weight gain is 25 to

35 pounds

BMI 25 - 29.9 is considered to be overweight; recommended weight gain is 15 to 25 pounds

BMI >30 is considered obese: recommended weight gain is 11 to 20 pounds.

The above weight gain applies to a singleton pregnancy; only one baby in the uterus.

Weight gain during pregnancy can be a very sensitive subject. Everyone seems to want to chime in and add their two cents. I commonly have patients coming in concerned that they don't look "big enough," or that they seem to be "further along" than their weeks gestation due to weight issues. Most OB/GYNs worth their salt will let you know if you need to reel it in a bit regarding weight gain during pregnancy. As for not gaining enough weight, per comments from the sometimes hyper-critical mommy peanut gallery, as long as baby is growing appropriately (likely determined by a growth ultrasound), no worries, it just means that you'll have fewer pounds to shed post-delivery.

Speaking of weight, I can't stress enough the importance of rockin' a healthy diet and exercising during pregnancy. It really pays off in the long run whether it's helping to decrease the risk of cesarean section and hypertensive disorders or staving off diabetes both during the pregnancy and later on in life. Not to mention the impact of a healthy diet and exercise on baby.

When to start PNVs (prenatal vitamins)?

If I've said it once I'll say it again, and I'll keep shouting it as many times as need be: The best time to start a prenatal vitamin is before you are pregnant! Initiating your prenatal vitamin regimen preconception ensures that your body has all those essentials during organogenesis, or that critical stage when baby's organ systems are developing. It may also deter the nausea that's often experienced in the first trimester.

What can the color of my urine tell me about my hydration status?

Mamas of the world, I empower you to HYDRATE! I'm always interested in the color of your urine as it is a pretty good indicator of your hydration status, though occasionally I'm thrown, as some prenatal vitamins tend to make urine darker. OB/GYNS want to see urine that is light yellow, not dark like tea. Being in a state of dryness makes for an unhappy uterus and may lead to cramping and contractions. Not drinking enough water can also lead to constipation, which can lead to abdominal pain and cramping.

In addition, drinking more water helps the kidneys do their job more effectively and efficiently. It helps in detoxing the body, while at the same time decreasing the likelihood of urinary tract infections and kidney stones.

Other benefits of increased water intake include less fatigue, greater mental alertness, as well as improved skin. Can we say stretch marks and acne?

I totally get it. Drinking a lot of water can, well, be a lot! I mean, you already have a baby tap dancing on your bladder, which makes you have to go constantly, and now this. Drinking more water is going to make you have to go to the bathroom even more (you may already be wondering how that's possible. #pregnantlife). Just consider it as taking one for the team. The pros of staying adequately hydrated during your pregnancy far outweigh the cons.

CHAPTER 2
ACHES, PAINS, AND OTHER "ANNOYANCES" OF PREGNANCY

How long will the nausea and vomiting last?

Too long! No, really, this is one thing about being pregnant that drove me bananas. I felt as if I started with the nausea immediately upon conceiving. Seriously, as soon as we found out we were pregnant, the nausea began, and while some folks may have just rumbly tummies, it didn't stop there with me. I had the double whammy of nausea and vomiting. Needless to say, this did a number on my teeth (more on that later). That feeling of queasiness, of not being able to eat anything, and even the slightest of smells making your stomach do cartwheels is not fun.

No one really knows what causes the nausea and vomiting associated with pregnancy, although the medical community has speculated that hormones (whether it be the estrogen levels, which are through the roof, or the spike in HCG, more commonly known as the pregnancy hormone) cause them. There are other conditions, such as molar pregnancies, that can be associated with nausea and vomiting, but we're not going to focus on those as this is all about normal pregnancies.

So, now that I've told you that no one really knows the cause of nausea and vomiting in pregnancy, I can at least tell you what I recommend to combat them. First, be comforted by the fact that these symptoms won't last forever (for most women anyway, it pretty much did last the entire pregnancy for me), usually they resolve once you get past the first trimester. Solutions I often recommend for relief include eating small, frequent meals. Soda crackers at the bedside are a must-have first thing in the morning. It's always a good idea to put something in your stomach upon rising and shining. I found this to be most helpful.

Ginger is also a good thing, but please don't go out and buy real ginger root. It's excessively strong. Things such as ginger ale, ginger snaps, or ginger candies will do. Other helpful pointers might be to eat your food at room temperature, avoid fatty or spicy foods, and try not to lie down immediately after eating. Another personal favorite is eating your favorite childhood cereal dry! The carbs are quite helpful in dealing with the nausea and vomiting of pregnancy. My usual recommendation is to snack on dry cereal throughout the day. Lucky Charms and Fruity Pebbles, anyone?

Is vaginal discharge normal during pregnancy?

A resounding YES! The amount of discharge you have will actually increase as your pregnancy progresses. My general rule of thumb where discharge is concerned is the following: As long as it doesn't itch, burn, or smell bad, it's likely normal.

Throw a panty liner on (honestly, I'm not sure why Tampax, Kotex, or Always haven't come out with a brand of panty liners made exclusively for pregnancy) to absorb this extra moisture, and change it frequently as the discharge can serve as a vulvar irritant.

Is nipple discharge normal during pregnancy?

As if the weight gain, back pain, swollen feet, and nausea weren't bad enough, now leaking breasts on top of all of that!

Got milk?

Nipple discharge in pregnancy is pretty par for the course. Most women will notice it in the second trimester, though some may experience it as early as the first. Your body, at this point, is raging with regard to its hormone levels.

The official term for this nipple discharge is colostrum. Pre-milk, if you will. It begins as thick and yellowish in color but gradually becomes clearer as you approach delivery. It provides all the key nutrients for baby until your milk finally comes in.

You may notice an increase in nipple discharge with breast stimulation or massage. I don't know about you, but my breasts were so tender during the course of my pregnancy that there was no massaging going on over here! Frankly, being attached to my pregnancy breasts was like an out of body experience for me, I went from an A cup to a solid B cup. For those of us that have small chests, this is usually one of the benefits of pregnancy.

There will be other changes as well. Your breasts and nipples becoming larger and darker, your areola becoming darker, the glands in your areola becoming prominent to the point of looking like little bumps, and did I mention that your décolletage may look like a road map due to the prominence of all the veins that seem to have miraculously appeared on your chest?

Is back/pelvic pressure normal during pregnancy?

Pelvic pressure during the latter part of a pregnancy, specifically during the last four weeks or so, is entirely normal as baby descends into the pelvis in preparation for making its entry into the world.

My first trimester ladies commonly ask me about cramping experienced during the initial phase of pregnancy. As long as there is no associated bleeding, this too, is par for the course.

Be mindful of things such as constipation and urinary tract infections, which can be causes of pelvic pressure. BIG PLUG for water consumption here! We seem to forget about the bowels in all of this. Constipation and bowel dysfunction is a very common cause of abdominal and pelvic pain in general, even in the non-pregnant state. With that said, water is your friend and will help counteract some of the slowing caused by the hormones of pregnancy, keeping you more regular. That and perhaps a stool softener (I like Colace), and/or Citrucel.

Although we routinely dip your urine at prenatal visits to look for any number of things, you will know the signs of a urinary tract infection if you experience them (pressure, frequency, urgency). If you feel as if this is happening to you, please let your OB/GYN know.

For those of you with jobs requiring you to stand on your feet for extended periods of time, the feeling of pressure is not going to be so farfetched. Consider gravity -- when you are standing for such prolonged periods, where is all the pressure? Do me a favor, look down.

Pressure in and of itself doesn't raise my eyebrows too much unless accompanied by some other findings. Those findings include a change in vaginal discharge from thick and mucousy to thin and watery, bleeding, or cramps that are getting progressively worse in terms of frequency and intensity.

What is round ligament pain?

ANNOYING at best! No, really, round ligament pain is one of those pregnancy pains that occurs during the second trimester. It can be sharp, dull, and occur on one or both sides of your pelvis/abdomen.

What causes it?

The round ligaments are the suspensory ligaments of your uterus; they are ligaments and bands of tissue flanking your uterus that connect it to your pelvic side walls. Now imagine that your uterus, which is normally about the size of your fist, has two rubber bands attached on either side of it. As it increases in mass with the progression of the pregnancy from the size of, say, an apple, to the size of a watermelon at full term, what happens to those ligaments (rubber bands, if you will) on the sides of your uterus? They stretch and are put under tension. Cue that bothersome pain. Round ligament pain can be aggravated by standing on your feet too long, certain positioning, and quick sudden motions such as rising too quickly. Taking a breather and getting off your feet might help relieve this pain. Uterine support belts can help take some of the pressure off these sensitive ligaments. And though many pregnant moms like to avoid taking any extra meds during the course of their pregnancy, Tylenol may provide some relief here.

What can I do about the swelling in my hands and legs? Is swelling during pregnancy normal?

Swelling during pregnancy is normal and will likely be noticed by you starting in the latter part of the second trimester/early part of the third trimester. The body requires an increase in fluid volume to support and maintain the growing pregnancy; swelling is a natural result of this.

You have probably noticed that swelling varies depending on the time of day and/or weather conditions. It may be worse at the end of the day as opposed to the beginning, or worse on hot days as opposed to cooler ones. You will also note that swelling tends to be worse in those "dependent" parts of your body, like hands, fingers, ankles, feet. Remember we had that conversation about gravity earlier? Same principle here. Where are your hands, fingers, ankles, and feet in relation to your body? Exactly! They are hanging down.

Something that may help reduce this irritating swelling is drinking plenty of water. Hmmmm… haven't we heard that somewhere before? And yet another benefit of drinking water during pregnancy reveals itself. As counterintuitive as this may sound, increasing your water intake will help decrease swelling by ridding your body of any toxins and extra salt, which may be contributing factors. Support hose and stockings may also reduce swelling by helping to increase circulation and fluid return from your lower extremities. Suggesting this during the summer months, particularly in New Jersey (hello extreme heat and humidity!) is almost laughable, but still an option. You make the call. As a note, these old-school support apparatuses also come in knee-high versions.

Being mindful of your salt intake can help reduce swelling, too, as well as getting off your feet and propping them up. Though this may prove to be difficult for some, avoiding prolonged periods on your feet will help to decrease the amount of pooling in your lower extremities. Sleeping on your left side will help avoid uterine compression of your interior vena cava (the major vessel that is responsible for blood flow return to your heart).

Once upon a time swelling was considered a hallmark finding of preeclampsia (more on this to come). By definition, preeclampsia is diagnosed by hypertension plus a certain amount of protein in your urine. Because most women experience swelling during pregnancy, it is no longer considered as part of the diagnostic criteria.

Why do my back/hips/pelvis hurt?

Your body is experiencing something pretty phenomenal in the form of a growing human inside your uterus! To accommodate this, the hormones of pregnancy have adjusted themselves to cause lots of relaxing and loosening of various bones, ligaments, and joints.

Let's start with your back. Your entire center of gravity begins to shift as your uterus grows and makes its appearance outside the pelvis, that is, above your pubic symphysis (that bone in the region of your bladder). For those of you whose physicians measure fundal height, aka uterus size and growth, at your prenatal visits, this is the landmark that we measure from. From here to the top of your uterus, or fundus. For the sake of reference, your uterus is typically at the level of the pubic symphysis at ten weeks gestation, halfway between your pubic symphysis and belly button at about 16 weeks gestation, and at the level of your belly button at 20 weeks gestation. As your uterus continues to grow, and you start to get that pregnant appearance, the stress on your lower back gets greater and greater. Let's not forget about the impact this has on your hips and pelvis, which stop being static and become more dynamic, or loosey-goosey, due to the hormones of pregnancy.

Whenever my pregnant moms mention the discomfort or pain they are experiencing in their lower back, hips or pelvis, I always, in my most sincere voice, tell them that I wish this were going to get better. Instead, as the pregnancy progresses, specifically as you enter into the latter stages of the third trimester, this discomfort will increase due to the laxity of the joints and ligaments in the hips and pelvis as they adjust to accommodate baby as he/she prepares to traverse the birthing canal.

Remember your mom telling you as a kid to "stand up straight?" You know, chin up, shoulders back, buttocks tucked. Well, during pregnancy, with your uterus growing larger and larger, sticking further and further out, the curvature of and stress on your lower back becomes greater and greater, making said request next to impossible. Uterine support belts are helpful in dealing with this pain as well as things such as putting a pillow in your seat for lower back support when sitting at your desk or driving. This is also a good reason to treat yourself to some prenatal massages.

Why don't my shoes fit anymore?

There were no "pumps and a bump" over here! I think that song is a throwback by MC Hammer. And no, I'm sure he wasn't talking about pregnancy. Seriously, I think I stopped wearing my high heels well into the first trimester of my pregnancy. I replaced them with more comfortable footwear, for me that included brands such as Clarks, Bjorns, and Danskos. No offense to these particular shoemakers, but let's just call a spade a spade; these aren't the usual suspects in a fashionable woman's wardrobe.

With the increase in fluid volume, the loosening of bones, joints, and ligaments (all attributed to the hormones of pregnancy), and your feet being in the most dependent portion of your body, this translates into widening and swelling. It's no wonder that your normal shoes don't fit anymore. Bring on the Hush Puppies and flip-flops.

What's the dark line down my abdomen?

That dark line between your belly button and your pubic bone would be your linea nigra. Not to fear, this line, which typically appears well into the second trimester, around week 23, will disappear after pregnancy. Truth be told, it has actually been there all along. The hormones of pregnancy are responsible for it becoming more noticeable. Such pigmentation changes, like darkening of the areola (area around your nipples), are more pronounced in darker skinned individuals.

What can I do about constipation?

Constipation is never any fun, pregnant or not. Those blasted hormones of pregnancy seem to wreak havoc on every bodily system, why would your bowels be any exception?

My favorite recommendations for dealing with constipation during pregnancy are simple. Once again, water, water, and more water. Not only will it keep you hydrated, but it will also combat constipation.

Another of my favorite recommendations is Colace. Yes, this can be purchased over the counter and it is a stool softener. Citrucel, another over the counter remedy (get the citrus flavor), was a mainstay in helping to keep me regular during my own pregnancy. Avoiding constipation is important during pregnancy as it is a very common cause of lower abdominal and pelvic pain, as well as hemorrhoids.

Are these large veins in my legs/labia normal?

YES! I can't begin to tell you how many emergency trips to the office I've seen for pregnant moms with lumps, bumps, and ginormous "things" on their vulvas that they weren't clearly able to describe but sure as hell were certain weren't normal. Upon further investigation by yours truly, we were able to discern that their vulva, which used to be the size of, let's say Massachusetts, but is now the size of, let's go with Texas, is entirely normal, and those humongous veins that seem to have appeared out of nowhere are typical varicosities of pregnancy. Unbeknownst to many, these super-sized veins don't just appear in your legs but can also show up in the region of your vulva. Think of where the legs, feet, and vulva are located. If they become painful or too uncomfortable, just as in the lower extremities where we recommend support stockings and hose, there are also vulvar supports for such circumstances during pregnancy. They're like jock straps for women. Oh, joy! Just know that these things do exist should the need arise.

What can I do about hemorrhoids?

Hemorrhoids. Yet ANOTHER gem of pregnancy! For most women, pregnancy will be their first experience with hemorrhoids. By definition, they are nothing more than varicose veins of the rectum which can occur due to the normal increase in fluid volume associated with pregnancy, pressure from an enlarging uterus, constipation (which leads to straining at the time of bowel movements) and pushing during labor and delivery.

Hemorrhoids can be painful, itchy, and sometimes cause rectal bleeding. The biggest recommendation to treat and prevent these common nuisances of pregnancy is to avoid constipation altogether. This can be accomplished by drinking plenty of water, consuming a diet that is fiber rich, and using a stool softener like Colace.

If you have already been struck with hemorrhoids and need symptom relief, common over the counter treatments such as witch hazel pads, TUCKS, ice packs, or certain hemorrhoid creams are often times safe for use. If you are unsure, just consult your OB/GYN.

How can I stop itching during pregnancy?

Remember, your skin is the largest organ of your body. I mention this only to highlight all the accommodating skin does to stretch with and support the bodily changes that occur as a result of pregnancy. Enlarged breasts and uterus sound familiar, girls?

Staying hydrated will help the skin stay moisturized and better lend itself to much needed elasticity. Soft and moist is better for stretching than dry and brittle.

I'm pretty old-school regarding my recommendations for maintaining moist, supple skin. I don't think you need to spend lots of money on lotions, potions, and elixirs promising miracle cures and preventative measures for things like stretch marks. As previously stated, drinking plenty of water is a HUGE help when maintaining moist and elastic skin during pregnancy, as well as use of heavy moisturizers such as shea or cocoa butter. These are easy, cheap, and guess what, AMAZING topical hydrators. Water and natural body butters were mainstays of treatment for soft, glowing skin during my own pregnancy. Moreover, while there is no magic remedy to prevent stretch marks during pregnancy, I used these techniques during my pregnancy and avoided stretch marks altogether.

Other helpful hints to keep the skin moisturized and stave off itching include things like maintaining a healthy diet. Remember, you are what you eat. Avoiding tight clothing, enjoying showers and baths that are not too hot, and using non-scented soaps (things with perfumes may serve as irritants to the skin) are all good recommendations.

Any itching that doesn't resolve with the aforementioned measures, gets progressively worse, or involves a rash of any kind warrants evaluation by your OB/GYN. There are certain conditions that can pose serious risks to your baby where itching is the hallmark symptom. Cholestasis of pregnancy is one such condition that immediately comes to mind.

What causes heartburn during pregnancy?

Yes, the hormones of pregnancy. We've already discussed the slowing effect that said hormones have on the digestive tract, including causing the valve that separates the stomach from the esophagus to relax. When this occurs, as is the case in pregnancy, the gastric juices that are a normal part of the digestive process gain access to the esophagus, causing the heartburn that is so characteristic of pregnancy. The other major culprit is a growing uterus that continues to shift things upwards as the pregnancy progresses.

Much of the same recommendations for treating nausea and vomiting in pregnancy hold true for good ole heartburn. You remember them. Small frequent meals, avoiding foods that are obvious triggers; i.e., spicy, fried, fatty. Avoiding foods with high acidity. Not consuming foods shortly before bedtime. Smooth/liquidy foods are also less likely to cause heartburn; soup, smoothie, shake, yogurt, pudding anyone? Tums is a common over the counter remedy commonly used for heartburn relief. If it feels as if you're consuming half the bottle in order to get relief, we should probably try something else. Let your OB/GYN know if these "go to" recommendations aren't cutting it. We've got a few other tricks up our sleeves to defeat this common pregnancy annoyance.

CHAPTER 3
FIRST TRIMESTER BLEEDING

There are times when being an OB/GYN isn't quite as amazing as one might think, specifically when you, the OB/GYN in question, happens to be pregnant! There is such a thing as knowing too much.

I swear, I feel for all the pregnant moms and patients out there who have experienced some sort of bleeding or spotting. There is no more anxiety-creating situation during a pregnancy. My entire first trimester, I tried not to think about being pregnant. I remember my partner/colleague/friend/OB/GYN commenting on how disconnected she thought I was concerning my own pregnancy. I wasn't, it was just that I wanted to, and thought I had to be, SUPER careful. Every time I went to the bathroom and wiped, I was afraid that I would see pink or light red. While I knew I was in great shape and had no real risk factors other than being old (I was over 35), I worried something would happen. Maybe I would miscarry. Who knows? All I knew was that I didn't want to become too attached to the pregnancy. Just in case.

While I know I often tell my pregnant moms not to worry or lose too much sleep about seeing light pink or a little bit of spotting during the early part of a pregnancy, believe me, I understand. I get it. Just keep the faith!

I had a small amount of spotting/bleeding, what does that mean?
In my best Charlie Brown exclamation as Lucy pulls the football away in his grave attempt to finally kick it, AAUGH!

Take a breath, calm down, and breathe. I always tell my patients, don't freak out until you see me totally spaz out, and that rarely, if ever, happens. At least not in front of you.

Ok, here we go. There are MANY common causes of first trimester bleeding. Some of them so commonplace that you may not even think to consider them. First, it might mean nothing. I know, I know. You're probably saying, "What do you mean it's nothing? I'm newly pregnant, bleeding, spotting, nervous, and scared, dammit!"

While it MIGHT be nothing, it could be SOMETHING as well. Something like a threatened abortion, an ectopic pregnancy, or signs of an abnormal pregnancy. I know the above phrases may seem a bit scary to you, but let's break it down.

Common causes of first trimester bleeding/spotting:

Implantation bleeding: This is more common than you think and is often times mistaken as that very light period you had. This typically occurs 10 to 14 days after conception.

Trauma: Once you become pregnant, everything becomes super vascular, that is, bleeds very easily. In my practice, the Pap smear, as well as testing for gonorrhea and chlamydia, are part of the new OB visit. The cervix, which is now SUPER vascular, can readily bleed when obtaining the Pap smear. I always counsel my patients not to freak out if they see a small amount of bleeding after this particular visit as it is not uncommon to have some light bleeding or spotting after this routine procedure. This alone saves a lot of worry and concern, as I know how the sight of blood affects pregnant moms -- it FREAKS THEM OUT!

Speaking of procedures, I did just mention that we obtain cultures testing for the presence of gonorrhea and chlamydia. Infection, such as, but not limited, to the aforementioned, is also a common cause of bleeding.

With the cervix being as vascular as it is in the newly pregnant state, bleeding post-sex is also a common cause of first trimester bleeding.

Threatened abortion: Any bleeding more significant than spotting is considered a threatened abortion until proven otherwise. No one wants to hear this. In any of my patients with vaginal bleeding, I bring them in immediately for a vaginal exam to see if there is an obvious source of the bleeding. I also look to see if the cervix is open or closed as an open cervix would be more indicative of an impending miscarriage or, more simply put, pregnancy loss.

I usually have an ultrasound done on patients with bleeding to see if there is an obvious source that might be seen on-screen. One of the more common findings is a subchorionic hemorrhage. A subchorionic hemorrhage is a collection of blood between the membranes of the placenta and the uterus. If this is detected on ultrasound, both its size and location are noted. While a subchorionic bleed can be associated with such things as preterm labor or miscarriage, in most cases they spontaneously resolve on their own. Follow-up ultrasounds are typically performed to assess for resolution or expansion. If you have been diagnosed with one of these, know that your bleeding will persist as long as the condition is present. This is typically characterized by bleeding and/or spotting that ranges from bright red to dark red to brown to no further bleeding once the subchorionic bleed has resolved. As an aside, the dark red to brownish color is usually indicative of old blood.

Ectopic Pregnancy: An ectopic pregnancy is any pregnancy outside the uterus. As I mentioned earlier, at the establish OB visit, the main objective is to ensure that there is indeed a pregnancy INSIDE the uterine cavity. Ectopic pregnancies can be associated with light bleeding and/or spotting and are obstetric emergencies that can be handled either medically or surgically depending on size, location, and the stability of the expectant mother.

Molar Pregnancy: On rare occasions, an abnormal mass develops inside the uterus instead of the normal fetus that typically results from the union of sperm and egg.

CHAPTER 4
VACCINATIONS DURING PREGNANCY

Is it ok to get the flu shot during pregnancy?
ABSO-FREAKING-LUTELY!

Along with recommendations for bundling up and staying warm, which surprisingly enough is usually not an issue during pregnancy, come strong suggestions for vaccinations, like the influenza vaccination in pregnant patients. October to May is designated as flu season. ACOG - (The American College of Obstetrics and Gynecology) recommends that all pregnant women, regardless of gestational age, receive the inactivated influenza vaccine. DON'T GET THE NASAL PREPARATION of the influenza vaccine as it is a live virus!

Why should I get the influenza vaccine?
Pregnancy increases a woman's risk of serious illness if she contracts the flu. Getting the flu shot during pregnancy provides some protection to the newborn baby via passive immunization. This becomes particularly important, as babies aren't eligible to receive the flu vaccine until they are at least six months of age. The take home message here is if not for you, do it for your unborn baby! Get your flu vaccine!

When should I get the Tdap vaccine?
The fact that we're asking when you need to get it is a clear indication that you should get it.

The Tdap (tetanus, diphtheria, and pertussis) vaccine, while it can be given at any time during pregnancy or during the postpartum period, should optimally be given between 27 and 36 weeks gestation in order to maximize maternal antibody response and ensure adequate passive newborn antibody transfer and levels. This becomes increasingly important since most of the morbidity and mortality associated with whooping cough occurs in infants less than three months of age.

Pregnant moms, family members, and caregivers (grandparents included) who will have close contact with newborns should get the Tdap vaccine as well. Newborns rely on the passive immunization they receive from vaccinated mothers. This is particularly important since newborns can't begin the pertussis vaccination series until two months of age.

What vaccinations are safe during pregnancy?

Ideally, we would love all pregnant women to be current on vaccinations pre-pregnancy, which is why I encourage women to get pre-conception counseling visits. This visit is aimed at making sure that a woman is in optimum condition to endure and maintain a pregnancy. It is at this visit that we go over immunization records, medical and surgical history, review medications to see what will or won't be safe during pregnancy, and address habits to improve pregnancy outcomes, such as weight loss and smoking cessation.

Okay mamas, time for a quick and easy breakdown on vaccines:

Hepatitis A/B:

Can be given before/during/after pregnancy if indicated.

Inactivated vaccine.

HPV (Human Papilloma Virus):

Can be given before/after pregnancy if criteria for receiving the vaccine are met (under age 26).

Inactivated vaccine.

Not currently given during pregnancy.

Influenza Vaccine:

The inactivated form of this vaccine can be given before/during/after pregnancy.

MMR (Measles/Mumps/Rubella):

If determined to be rubella non-immune during the pregnancy, can be given postpartum.

If determined to be rubella non-immune pre-pregnancy, can be given before pregnancy. It is, however, recommended that one wait four weeks before attempting conception.

Live vaccine.

CANNOT be given during pregnancy.

Meningococcal/Pneumococcal:

Inactivated vaccines.

Can be given before/during/after pregnancy if indicated.

Tdap:

Toxoid/inactivated vaccine.

Can be given before/during/after pregnancy if indicated.

Varicella:

Live vaccine.

CANNOT be given during pregnancy.

If determined to be varicella non-immune during the pregnancy, the vaccine can be given postpartum.

If determined to be varicella non-immune (having never had the chicken pox) pre-pregnancy, the vaccine can be given before pregnancy. It is however, as with the MMR vaccine, recommended that one wait four weeks before attempting to conceive.

CHAPTER 5
TRAVEL DURING PREGNANCY

Can I travel during pregnancy?

Strap up, globetrotter, because I say heck yeah! Pregnancy is no reason to be all cooped up in the house or limited to walks around the mall or neighborhood park. Whether it be by plane, train, or automobile, as long as there are no issues with the pregnancy, and you've gotten approval from your OB, you should be good to go.

When can I no longer fly? What are your recommendations?

When you can no longer fly, or if you will even be permitted to fly, will largely depend on the course of your pregnancy. If you have a pregnancy that is considered high risk, whether that be due to common problems such as gestational diabetes, high blood pressure, bleeding, multiple gestation, or preterm labor and contractions, your obstetrician may be a bit hesitant to allow you to travel too far outside of your hospital radius.

The answer to this question may also depend on the airline. Carriers have varying guidelines on travel during pregnancy, sometimes restricting expectant moms based on their gestational age. This may differ depending on whether the intended travel is domestic or international, and more specifically how close to the due date the pregnant passenger is. Depending on the woman's gestational age, a letter from her physician as well as clearance from the airlines special coordinator may be required. You would be wise to check with your specific airline, as there is no blanket policy for air travel. For most, recommendations for the latest gestational age one should travel vary from 32 to 36 weeks.

For those patients who are traveling, no matter how near or far, I always advise traveling with a copy of your prenatal record. Your obstetrician's office should have no problem providing this. Having a copy of your prenatal record is paramount as it provides an overview of your pregnancy up to your current gestation and contains all the pertinent highlights of your pregnancy.

Specifically, your lab work, ultrasound findings, problems, and management up to said point. It's like an AmEx for your baby: Don't leave home without it!

What is the two-hour stationary rule in travel?

If you are going to be stationary for more than two hours at a time, whether you are flying, driving, or riding on a train, I always advise getting up, taking a walk up and down the aisles, or frequent visits to rest stations. If you are not in a position to ambulate, leg exercises will do. Try flexing and extending your feet and rotating them in circular motions both clockwise and counterclockwise.

The reasoning behind this recommendation is to avoid the increased risk of clotting that exists as a result of being pregnant.

CHAPTER 6
DUE DATE

When is my due date?

Your due date, also known as your EDC (estimated date of confinement) or EDD (estimated date of delivery) is the gestational age at which the onset of labor is expected to spontaneously occur. In weeks gestation, this is usually the 40-week mark.

While there are numerous ways to arrive at the EDC/EDD, Naegele's Rule remains a personal favorite. It states that we can determine the due date by adding a year, subtracting three months, and adding seven days to the first day of a woman's last menstrual period. For example, let's say your last menstrual period was October 10, 2014. According to Naegele's Rule, your due date would be July 17, 2015. Although Naegele's Rule is a bit old-school by most standards, you've heard me say it enough already: I LOVE OLD-SCHOOL! It's a quick and easy way for me to approximate a due date, especially since the first question I'm usually asked by super excited moms and parents-to-be is, "WHEN'S THE DUE DATE?"

I was able to determine the due date of my own daughter using Naegele's Rule. My periods were as guaranteed as the old-school postal service (what did they used to say, something about through rain, snow, and sleet?). Anyway, we knew the EXACT date of conception and using Naegele's Rule we handpicked the day she would be delivered by C-section.

While Naegele's Rule is a quick and easy way to determine the due date, when I see patients for an establish pregnancy visit, the main purpose of the appointment is for me to determine not only a due date, but also how far along into the pregnancy the expectant mother currently is. This is most commonly accomplished by obtaining an ultrasound measurement known as a crown-rump length.

A crown-rump length is a measurement typically obtained by transvaginal ultrasound and looks at the distance between the crown, or head, and the rump, or buttocks, of the fetus. In my practice, in a woman with a known last menstrual period, we typically use the due date determined by the last menstrual period. The crown-rump length measurement is used more for confirmatory purposes. If, however, there is more than a week's discrepancy, a seven-day difference between the date obtained using the last menstrual period and that obtained using the crown-rump length, we go with the dating determined using the crown-rump length.

Got it? Hoping I didn't lose you on that one.

More simply put, as long as the dating is congruent, we use the dating obtained by last menstrual period; if there is more than a seven-day discrepancy in the dating obtained by the aforementioned methods, we go with the dating determined by using the crown-rump length measurement.

When is it safe to tell family and friends I'm pregnant?

How about WHENEVER YOU WANT TO!

The most common reason for not telling is the risk of miscarriage. People are afraid to share the news of having a baby because they are afraid of having to deal with the aftermath in case of the unthinkable. Who wants to share the news of pregnancy only to miscarry and have to deal with the constant congrats for a pregnancy that is no more? Or, having to repeatedly explain what happened and that you are no longer pregnant?

On the flip side, how hard is it to keep something like a new pregnancy to yourself? If you are anything like me, I was literally bursting at the seams (yes, literally)! At the six-week mark I couldn't fit into any of my normal clothes and immediately had to resort to maternity wear. Being as petite as I am, it wasn't too hard to notice my "glow" or increase in breast size.

My always-in-your-business sister was the first to notice. We were planning to tell my parents over the weekend. My wife and I were meeting my family in Washington, D.C. for President Obama's inauguration. Upon first seeing me I remember my sister knowingly calling out to my father and brother, "Hey Dad, Donald, doesn't Ang look different to you somehow?" I remember my pops and brother saying no and that other than being my normally beautiful self, they didn't notice a difference (leave it to men not to notice the subtleties). With that response from my father and brother, my sister wandered over to my wife and I stating, "Ladies, we clearly have a lot of catching up to do!"

We didn't share our pregnancy news until we were outside of the first trimester. Our choice not to share included knowing that the risk of miscarriage, which is generally 15 percent overall, was slightly increased due to me being of advanced maternal age (greater than or equal to age 35). Please note, however, that the further along in gestation you progress during the first trimester, the lesser your chances are of miscarrying. For example, once a heartbeat is confirmed by ultrasound at the eight-week mark, the risk of miscarriage from that point on is roughly three percent.

The other reason we chose to wait to share our news is we weren't really sure how our families would react. My dad, after all, was and still is the pastor of one of the largest Baptist churches in Cincinnati. I knew it was already tough enough for him dealing with the fact that he had a lesbian daughter, and now his lesbian daughter and her wife were bringing a child into the world. While I have always marched to the beat of my own drum and learned a long time ago to follow my heart's desires, I am still very sensitive to how my actions may affect others.

While we were fortunate in that our pregnancy went off without a hitch, and we had the love and support of our family and friends, what would have happened if things hadn't turned out quite so well? Being able to rely on those same family and friends through a difficult time such as a miscarriage would certainly have proven to be beneficial.

My general rule of thumb is this: *Do what feels good for you and your partner.* There is no right or wrong answer here, no line drawn in the sand that says, "Today is the day to shout it to the world." Whenever you feel ready to invite others into your amazing journey, open the doors, sister. The same people that will support you in your joy are the same ones you may need to console you during your pain.

What happens if I go beyond my due date?

Contrary to popular belief, time doesn't stand still, and in most pregnancies, due dates can and will pass! Some of the more memorable things my expectant moms say, even around the 36-week mark, include phrases like, "I'm done!", "I'm so over this!", "Enough already!" I could go on and on. Just like those due dates. I TOTALLY GET IT! No one ever likes to admit this, and some (er, most) are afraid to even acknowledge this, so I'll just put it out there. PREGNANCY IS A REAL ASS-KICKER!

Back to the question at hand. I am asked this about due dates all the time. As beautiful as pregnancy is, it is not the most comfortable state of existence, what with all the heartburn, constipation, back pain, and sleepless nights. Because of this, most expectant mothers cannot wait to deliver baby.

So, what exactly does happen if you go beyond your due date? Honestly, not much. In my practice, once a mother reaches and exceeds her due date, we implement some form of antepartum testing, which usually includes an NST (non-stress test), and/or a BPP (biophysical profile). The purpose of the testing is to ensure that baby remains in a safe environment to continue with the pregnancy.

The non-stress test is easy to perform. It's our way of assessing fetal heart tones and looking at uterine activity. This is accomplished by connecting two belts around the gravid uterus and looking at the uterus. Non-stress testing lasts for at least 20 minutes. As long as this testing is reassuring, the pregnancy is safe to continue. And just what does "reassuring" look like or mean? The fetal heart tracing reveals fetal heart tones that show good beat-to-beat variability and accelerations or increases in baby's heart rate that are at least 15 beats above baseline and last for at least 15 seconds. If said criteria are not met, the next step is typically to proceed with a biophysical profile.

The biophysical profile is another test that is often utilized to assess a pregnancy that has gone beyond its due date. The biophysical profile is an ultrasound that looks at a couple of different parameters, including movement, tone, breathing, and amniotic fluid level. If the biophysical profile is reassuring, the pregnancy, once again, is safe to continue. Reassuring is defined by scoring an 8 out of 8. Each category, as noted above, is scored on a scale of 0 to 2. If the criteria for movement, breathing, tone, and amniotic fluid levels are met, a score of 2 is given to each. If these criteria are not met, a score of 0 is assigned.

Having gone beyond 40 weeks of gestation, if the antenatal testing, as mentioned above, is reassuring, the pregnancy is allowed to progress to 41 weeks. If by 41 weeks the expectant mother has not delivered, we typically pick a date for delivery whether that be via induction of labor or cesarean section. It is not our general practice to allow a pregnancy to go beyond 42 weeks gestation as the risks of remaining pregnant at this gestational age far exceed the safety of allowing the pregnancy to continue.

Just what are the risks associated with remaining pregnant beyond 42 weeks? An increase in perinatal morbidity and mortality for one. This translates into an increased risk of stillbirth and admission to the NICU (neonatal intensive care unit). A condition termed oligohydramnios, occurs when low amniotic fluid levels lead to umbilical cord compression during labor, which in turn can yield a non-reassuring or concerning fetal heart tracing. Increases in risks of cesarean section, macrosomia (large baby), meconium (baby having a bowel movement in utero), and aspiration syndrome are also seen in post-term pregnancies (ones that go beyond 42 weeks).

TMI? I know, it's a lot. (You can see why this OB/GYN was her own worst enemy while pregnant!) Take a beat, a deep breath, hug your belly, girl. It's time to get back into the fun stuff.

CHAPTER 7
PREGNANCY MILESTONES

Fetal movement. It's everything! It's one of the first good things that women experience during pregnancy. Prior to this it has been about nausea, vomiting, painful breasts, you know. Up to this point, the only real indicator that all is well was hearing fetal heart tones at your prenatal visits. We go from wondering if everything is okay to questioning whether or not that twinge, or flutter, was the baby moving to baby moving all the time! This is when the magic really begins.

When should I start feeling baby move?
This is different for everybody! Specifically, if you are a first-time mom versus a mom that has already experienced childbirth. "Quickening," as this is typically termed, is usually noted between 16 and 22 weeks, but I tell my new moms that it may take up to 20 or 22 weeks before you actually feel baby moving. For my ladies who have been through this before, some tell me they have felt fetal movement as early as 14 weeks.

You all know my favorite question to ask at the beginning of obstetric visits: "Is baby movin' and groovin'?" I usually don't even bother asking this until around 16 weeks, and when I do, it's with the slightest bit of hesitancy as it's still pretty early in the pregnancy. Often times I anticipate that the answer to the aforementioned question at such an early gestation is going to be a big fat N-O. And that's all gravy, baby.

The perception of fetal movement is super important because up until this point, most women aren't really connected to their pregnancies. We're still afraid of miscarrying, worrying about what that light pink discharge on the toilet paper really means, what our new bodies will look like, and if everything is truly okay. I mean, aside from the monthly prenatal visits that you have up to this point, there is no other obvious way to know if everything is progressing as expected. Technology why haven't you caught up with the female body yet? (Pfft, it's probably a man.)

I remember the early part of my own pregnancy and how my colleague, who was my doctor, talked about the weird dynamic we had. There's nothing stranger than having someone that you know on a personal level, are friends with, someone that isn't your spouse, be privy to the most intimate details of your health, and, to top it off, gets to see your vajayjay. Anyway, I remember my friend and colleague relaying to me how detached she thought I was about the whole pregnancy during the early stages. To be honest, it wasn't detachment, I just didn't know everything was "fine" until we got those heart tones by Doppler. I was like Whitney waiting to exhale but, finally, I could.

I remember the first time we felt our lovebug move. Given my profession, you wouldn't think that I would be so clueless, but I certainly was. First-time mom jitters definitely trumped OB/GYN expertise, let me tell you. I was sitting up in bed reading some fashion magazine while my other half was busy in the restroom doing her eyebrows. Suddenly, I felt something! I was truly taken by surprise. Then I felt it again! Being the Einstein that I am, I thought it was gas or something (as an aside, fetal movement is oft times described as a bubbly feeling or gas-like). I quickly called my wife to the bedside and asked her to take a look. For the record, my wife is not a physician, her background is in business, finance, leadership, fashion and design (yup, snagged a good one), so what medical expertise she was going to impart, I have no idea. Anyway, she felt my belly and said, "Baba, it's the baby!" We were 16 weeks along.

NEWSFLASH! I'm a board-certified obstetrician/gynecologist and even I wasn't sure what I was feeling that first time. So, don't feel bad or beat yourself up if you are unsure of whether or not you actually felt or are feeling something.

When will we be able to hear the baby's heartbeat with the Doppler?
Fetal heart tones are like music to your ears! I guarantee you it will be the best sound you ever hear. Even if I felt baby "movin' and groovin'," I couldn't be convinced that everything was okay until I heard that heartbeat. The earliest that I will even attempt to listen for fetal heart tones with my Doppler is ten weeks gestation. Prior to that, I typically use the ultrasound to document the presence of fetal heart tones.

Even after ten weeks I occasionally have difficulty getting heart tones with the Doppler. Talk about a look of sheer panic appearing on the faces of my expectant mothers! We all literally hold our breaths until we hear that familiar sound. Some of the obvious reasons I might have difficulty finding heart tones by Doppler include an anterior placenta---in other words, the placenta being in such a position that it sort of serves as a buffer to the Doppler listening device--- or the placenta gets in the way, so to speak. This isn't an issue once we progress further along in gestation. The other reason is that the baby is moving all over the place! I can't tell you how many times I've had to chase heart tones for minutes at a time.

If I still can't find heart tones, I yield to the ultrasound, which does the whole two birds one stone thing. One, I don't know a pregnant mom who doesn't love an opportunity to see her baby, and two, it's really easy for me to visualize heart tones.

When will we be able to determine the sex of the baby?

Once upon a time, the anatomy scan (ultrasound) that is performed at 18 to 20 weeks became a HUGE landmark in pregnancy as it typically revealed the moment when you could determine the sex of the baby. While the anatomy scan holds a totally different level of significance for the physician (it's the scan that allows visualization of all the important organ systems), most patients view this scan as nothing more than "the ultrasound that will let me know what I'm having." This always makes me smile, as personally, this is the least important bit of information obtained from this scan, at least from a medical point of view.

When it's time for your ultrasound, please keep in mind that being able to determine baby's gender via ultrasound is going to be dependent on whether or not baby is showing the goods, which isn't always the case. A newer method for determining fetal gender is called cell-free fetal DNA. This testing, often times classified as NIPT (noninvasive prenatal testing), can be done after ten weeks gestation. While it is typically used to screen for trisomies such as trisomy 21 (Down syndrome), 18 (Edwards syndrome), and 13 (Patau Syndrome), it can also be used to determine the sex of the baby by detecting and testing fetal cells found in the maternal bloodstream. Pretty freakin' cool, right? Okay, technology, you get a few points back in your column.

Being an obstetrician and all, as you can imagine, I had ready access to an ultrasound machine. My ultrasound technician at the time, and still to this day, is the best that I have EVER worked with. Believe me, she's got skills! Anyway, being the slightly erratic and impatient individual that I am, I decided to have an early ultrasound. Upon performing the scan, my wife and I were informed that we were having a boy. We left the office, went out for a cup of coffee---yes, I was consuming a grande soy caramel macchiato daily---and cried and cried and cried. What were we, two lesbians, very girly women, going to do with a boy? I mean, I had the sports down to a T, I can talk game with the best of 'em, but, with two moms like us the poor kid was sure to be gay (not that there's anything wrong with that, I mean, HELLO!)! So, we went on about our business, having accepted that which was meant/going to be, and proceeded with preparing for our son to arrive. We had his room painted and everything.

So, that original scan was done around 15 weeks or so. Fast forward to my regularly scheduled anatomy scan at 20 weeks. Same technician, same key players (my wife and I). As the scan is being performed, the room all of a sudden went dead silent! Now you have to remember, I'm not just your ordinary patient. While being scanned, I was doing my own assessment of things, noting the heart, brain, kidneys, and last but not least, THE GENITALIA. My wife, who had asked for our friend and ultrasonographer to take another look, kept asking, "What's wrong? Is everything okay?"
The first thing I did was reach for my cellphone, call our painter, and tell him he had to repaint the baby's room.
"WE'RE HAVING A GIRL!"
We were so excited. I share this tale to remind you of this, babies show when they want to show, and ultrasound is never 100 percent.

CHAPTER 8
TESTING IN PREGNANCY

Pregnancy is a really big deal, and there is a lot that goes into making sure you have a safe, healthy pregnancy. With all the testing that will be offered throughout the course of your journey, trying to figure out why certain assessments are being recommended and whether or not you should proceed with them can be overwhelming to say the least.

During my pregnancy experience, I found less to be more. My wife and my take on things, specifically regarding the screening tests, was, as our daughter often reminds us, "You get what you get and you don't get upset." That really is how we approached things. We opted out of all the screening tests and only proceeded with those that were necessary based on the course of our pregnancy. I'm hopeful that this chapter will direct you in making the most informed decisions for your current pregnancy. It will answer the whats, whens, and whys of all those pins, pricks, and pokes.

How many ultrasounds will I get during my pregnancy?

I so wish I knew the magic number, but honestly the answer to this question depends on several factors, ranging from how the pregnancy was conceived (was conception spontaneous or with assistance?) to what type of insurance you have (think coverage, ladies) to whether or not your current pregnancy is high or low risk to issues you or baby might be having at your current appointment.

For those of you that have a low risk, uncomplicated pregnancy---and what I mean by this is that you have no medical issues that may complicate the pregnancy, such as high blood pressure, diabetes, or multiple gestation (twins, triplets) --- you will typically have an ultrasound in the first trimester to establish dating and another ultrasound between 18 and 20 weeks. This scan is more commonly known as the anatomy scan, or as most patients call it, "the ultrasound where we get to find out the sex of the baby."

Now that's just two ultrasounds. That doesn't take into account ultrasounds that are a part of certain screening tests done in the first trimester where a nuchal translucency measurement is obtained. This is typically done between 11 and 13.6 weeks and is a screening test for Down syndrome and other chromosomal abnormalities. If the screening test comes back abnormal and further, definitive testing in the form of an amniocentesis or CVS, is necessary (no worries, we will get to these tests a bit later) more ultrasounds will be involved. In the event that you have a pregnancy that is complicated with something like, say, high blood pressure or diabetes (God forbid!), where things like placental function and growth of the baby are monitored very closely, then, you guessed it, there will be more ultrasounds.

In a nutshell, the number of ultrasounds that you will have in a given pregnancy is dependent on the risk associated with the pregnancy, as well as how the pregnancy is progressing in general.

How do you decide whether or not to get screening tests for Down syndrome and neural tube defects?
This question isn't nearly as difficult as we make it out to be. I remember being the patient and deciding whether or not I wanted any of the screening tests offered in my pregnancy for various chromosomal and genetic abnormalities. Because I was AMA (advanced maternal age), I was hyper aware during my pregnancy. And, no, we're not talking member of the American Medical Association, folks, but advanced maternal age, which is defined as being aged 35 or greater at the time of delivery. For the record, I was 37 when my daughter was born. Not only did I have the screening tests to consider, but the definitive testing options as well, an amniocentesis or CVS (chorionic villus sampling). My age, after all, put my baby at an increased risk for chromosomal and genetic abnormalities. When it came down to it, these are the factors that my wife and I considered when making the decision whether or not to have any testing done, and things I ask my patients to consider when electing for screening versus definitive testing to be performed.

Number one, recognize that the screening tests are just that, screening tests. If they come back abnormal you will have to have definitive testing done to confirm the initial results.

How will knowing these results affect your current pregnancy?

Will it affect whether or not you proceed with the pregnancy?

Will it help you to better cope/deal with a pregnancy if you know ahead of time that your pregnancy is affected with one of the trisomies, such as Down syndrome, or another chromosomal or genetic issue? Or, will it not affect anything at all, because regardless of the outcome of such testing, you are going to love and cherish the child beautifully bestowed upon you?

Number two, are there health and lifestyle factors that put you at an increased risk? Things like race, family history, previously affected children, and age.

There is no right or wrong answer here. Ultimately, it comes down to what you think is best for you. Personally speaking, and I always share with my patients that I didn't get any of the screening tests done, my risk factor was being "an old gal." Knowing all that I know as a board certified, obstetrician and gynecologist, I knew that outside of my age, I was healthy, had no significant family history, and that my wife and I would love our child unconditionally. Besides, I'm one of those folks that knowing ahead of time probably would have added more stress to my life and caused significant anxiety.

While this visit can be a bit daunting and overwhelming, to say the least, such issues are broached pretty early in the pregnancy, specifically with the initial screening test of a time-sensitive nuchal translucency (done between 11- and 13.6-weeks gestation). That way, there is plenty of opportunity to discuss and decide what will be best for you and your pregnancy.

Speaking of what tests to have or not to have, these are the major players to consider:

NTL (Nuchal translucency): As previously mentioned, this is a test performed via ultrasound and is done between 11 and 13.6 weeks. It is time-sensitive! This test is done by a specialist who performs a transabdominal ultrasound and measures the "nuchal fold," or, in layman's terms, the thickness of skin at the nape of baby's neck. Based on this measurement, as well as maternal blood testing where us docs look at several analytes produced by the placenta, specifically PAPP-A (pregnancy associated plasma protein) and HCG (human chorionic gonadotropin), we come up with a relative risk for the baby having Down syndrome or other chromosomal abnormalities.

Cell-Free Fetal DNA: This screening test is offered at the time of the nuchal translucency and can be performed any time after ten weeks gestation. This test is pretty sweet. It involves a maternal blood draw where fetal cells are detected in the mother's blood stream and screening for things such as Trisomy 13, 18, and 21 are performed. As an added bonus, we are also able to determine the sex of the baby. For those who are dying to know, you no longer have to wait until that 20-week anatomy scan. I often wonder if testing such as this will make things such as amniocentesis and CVS obsolete in the near future.

AFP (Alpha-Fetoprotein): This is another screening test that is performed in the second trimester, usually between 15 and 20 weeks, but ideally between 16 and 18 weeks. This screens for neural tube defects. Whenever you think neural tube, think brain and spinal cord. The neural tube defect that is most commonly known to you is probably spina bifida. This test also screens for abdominal wall defects.

Quad Screen: This screening test is performed in the second trimester, typically between 15 and 20 weeks. It's all about analysis of maternal blood. As suggested by the name, it looks at four markers, those being: AFP (alpha-fetoprotein), Inhibin, Estriol, and HcG (Human Chorionic Gonadotropin), the latter three being products of the placenta, the former being produced by the fetal liver. I like to consider this particular test one-stop shopping, if you will, as it screens for various chromosomal abnormalities as well as neural tube defects. So, if you happen to miss the deadline for any of the aforementioned testing, there is still this second trimester option if you are interested in having some sort of screening test done.

If my screening test comes back abnormal, then what?

YIKES!! This is every mother's worst nightmare!

First thing's first: Please keep in mind that this is only a screening test!! The purpose of screening tests is to determine if baby is at an increased risk for certain chromosomal abnormalities and/or birth defects. Also, as with any screening test, there can be false negatives, as well as false positives.

SO BREATHE, wooooooooosaaaaaah!

The next step is usually getting a detailed ultrasound to take a closer look at baby. In my realm, we used to call this a level II ultrasound, to keep it simple, we'll refer to it as a detailed anatomy scan that is typically done by a specialist, your friendly perinatologist, aka, high risk pregnancy doctor, aka MFM (maternal fetal medicine). Depending on which of the above screening tests have or have not been done, additional testing such as cfDNA, if not already done, may be offered. Consultation with a genetic counselor, depending on the finding, may also be warranted. Ultimately, you will be offered diagnostic testing such as an amniocentesis or CVS (chorionic villus sampling) depending on how far along you are in your pregnancy.

A little aside here, some women just skip the screening tests altogether and opt for one of these two tests. These tests are DEFINITIVE:

Amniocentesis: This is the diagnostic test that most of you have heard of or are most familiar with. It is done between 15 and 20 weeks gestation, typically by a specialist, and involves an ultrasound-guided removal of a sample of amniotic fluid via a needle that is inserted through the maternal abdomen and into the amniotic sac. This fluid in turn is sent off for analysis to detect chromosomal, genetic, and/or neural tube defects.

CVS (Chorionic Villus Sampling): This is the second form of prenatal diagnostic testing but one you are probably less familiar with. It is typically performed between ten and 12 weeks and is also done under ultrasound guidance (either vaginal or abdominal). It involves obtaining a sample of the placenta, which is then sent off for analysis for chromosomal and/or genetic abnormalities. Aside from the timing of when these tests are performed, it's important to note that CVS does not test for neural tube defects. Furthermore, additional testing, either via second trimester screening or amniocentesis, would have to be utilized to screen or test for such.

When do I get screened for gestational diabetes?

Typically, between 26 and 28 weeks gestation. However, if you are at an increased risk for developing gestational diabetes (you are overweight, have a family history of diabetes, have a history of delivering a large baby in a previous pregnancy, have previously been affected by gestational diabetes, or belong to any racial group other than Caucasian) you may be screened not only at the designated 26 to 28 weeks gestation, but earlier in the pregnancy, specifically, during the first trimester. If I have a patient that I feel is at an increased risk for developing gestational diabetes I will typically screen her at the time we draw her initial prenatal labs, as well as during the 26 to 28-week time frame.

We will talk about gestational diabetes in depth in another section, but allow me to say, this is the screening test I was least excited about performing. I used to always say, "If the good Lord ever wanted to get back at me, He would've made me a gestational diabetic." Getting blood drawn, getting stuck with needles... To be clear, I AM THE BIGGEST CHICKEN IN THE WORLD. I can't even imagine having to stick myself four times a day to check blood sugars. Let alone, rewind the tape, how about EVEN GETTING to the diagnosis, that one-hour screening glucola test, choose whatever flavor you desire (cola, orange, lemon lime), I found them all to be equally detestable. Though many of you have told me that you didn't mind the flavor so much, I could barely get it down. FORTUNATELY, I passed my one-hour screening test and didn't have to go for the diagnostic test -- dun, dun, dunnn: THE THREE-HOUR GLUCOSE TOLERANCE TEST!

I'm such a wimp.

But before we get to that, what do you need to know about the one-hour glucola test? It is a screening test for gestational diabetes (more on this to come) and looks at your body's ability to process sugar in the pregnant state. You DO NOT have to fast for this test, however, I don't recommend eating French toast for breakfast prior to going to the lab for evaluation. You will drink a sugary drink (flavor of your choice: cola, orange, lemon lime to name a few) and an hour later your blood will be drawn. The amount of sugar in your body will be measured in milligrams per deciliter. In my practice, we use 140mg/dl as the cut-off value. Anything above this prompts referral for the diagnostic test, which is the three-hour glucose tolerance test (GTT). Some other practices use 130 as the cut-off value.

If, indeed, you are referred for definitive testing in the form of a three-hour glucose tolerance test, you will drink yet another sugary drink, and four values will be measured. Fasting, one-hour, two-hour, and three-hour glucose levels. You will have met the diagnostic criteria for gestational diabetes if two or more values are abnormal. However, it is my general practice to recommend close monitoring via dietary recommendations and glucose measurements even in those patients having one abnormal value. Individuals meeting the criteria for gestational diabetes are sent for a nutrition and dietary consultation as well as instruction on how to properly measure their blood sugars. If we find that improved diet alone is not sufficient in maintaining adequate glucose control, an insulin agent may be added. It is the insulin-controlled diabetics that require more intense monitoring in the form of growth ultrasounds, and antepartum testing. Those with gestational diabetes well-controlled with diet alone typically don't require any additional antepartum surveillance.

I remember how I felt about getting this test done and then waiting for the results. I had the distinct advantage of being able to look up my own lab results. I repeatedly said the same thing to myself, asked God above, if He was listening: "PLEASE don't let me have gestational diabetes, PLEASE don't let me have gestational diabetes, PLEASE don't let me have gestational diabetes!"

SO, as soon as the results are back, I either notify you of the results, OR it's the first thing out of my mouth at your visit following testing.

Why do you take so much blood for my prenatal battery?

We are all secretly vampires! Ha, just kidding.

If you truly understood all the tests that comprise the prenatal battery, you would probably ask why we don't take a bit more. No, seriously, we test for a whole lot of things with the prenatal battery. Just for kicks and giggles, here are the tests that are included in the prenatal battery that I routinely order:

Type and screen
Antibody screen
Rubella status
Toxoplasmosis antibody status
Parvovirus antibody status
Complete blood count
Hepatitis B surface antigen status
Urine analysis
Cystic fibrosis
SMA (spinal muscular atrophy)
Fragile X syndrome
Hemoglobin electrophoresis
Thyroid function studies
HIV status

This list doesn't include the Pap smear or the screenings for gonorrhea and chlamydia that are also a part of the prenatal battery but obtained at the time of your overall exam.

What is group B strep?

GBS (group B strep) sounds pretty scary but is not a sexually transmitted infection. GBS is a bacterium that can dwell in our digestive tracts, urinary, or reproductive systems. Being part of our natural flora, it typically has no effect on our day-to-day living. We check for its presence in pregnant women because testing positive and spreading the bacteria from mother to baby can have some pretty serious consequences, the most common issues being lung infection, blood infection, and meningitis.

When do you test for group B strep and why is it important?

We typically test for GBS between 35 and 37 weeks of pregnancy. I always give patients a heads up when obtaining this culture as it involves obtaining a swab from inside the vagina, down the perineum (the skin between the opening of the vagina and the rectum), and a poke in the rectum. Nobody likes that sort of surprise!

If you test positive for GBS it just means that you'll be treated with antibiotics during the course of your labor to prevent its spread to baby. If you have had a previous infant affected by GBS, or have a positive urine culture for GBS during your current pregnancy, you are already considered to be colonized and will not need further cultures but will be treated automatically.

What are fetal kick counts?

Whenever I say this or even think about the phrase, I imagine babies playing soccer inside the uterus. I know, just something else to add to my bizarreness, which, frankly, is one of my more endearing attributes. Once I finally figured out that the flutters, and gas pains, were my daughter rolling around inside of me, I realized she was quite the mover and shaker. She kept me up all the time! As a result of how much my mini-me moved when she was inside my uterus, we call her Fish, a well-deserved nickname as she was all over the place back then, and continues to be in the outside world. No surprise she turned out to be an amazing swimmer. I always say, activity in utero translates to activity outside of the uterus. So, if your baby is a busy body on the inside, get ready to be busy when he or she is born!

Fetal kick counts are ways for moms to assess fetal well-being. As a pregnancy progresses, an expectant mother will gradually learn baby's activity cycles, that is, when baby is most active and when baby sleeps. (Yes, those little seeds have routines even before they hit the real world.) Performing fetal kick counts is fairly easy and should be done daily, though I don't recommend initiating them until 28 weeks gestation.

I advise each of my moms to go into a quiet room and either lay on her left side or find a position that is most comfortable for her. Next comes the kick counting. While there are numerous methods to count kicks, one of the more standard, easy to remember methods is seeing how long it takes to feel ten discrete fetal movements. Those movements can be kicks, punches, cartwheels, or rolls. One of the methods approved by The American College of Obstetrics and Gynecologists (ACOG) is the ten kicks within two hours protocol. Most will find that they are able to perceive ten fetal movements in much less time than two hours, which is great! If, however, for any reason, you have concerns about signs of fetal movement, lack thereof, or if fetal kick counts aren't met, you should IMMEDIATELY contact your doctor.

NST/BPP, why do we get them? What do they tell us?

I know, it feels like the testing never ends, right? I hated it (self-admitted wuss over here). But these ain't too bad. Promise.

The non-stress test (NST) and biophysical profile (BPP) are examples of antepartum testing. More simply put, they are tests that can be implemented at various stages of pregnancy to assess fetal well-being, specifically in pregnancies that are at an increased risk for fetal death. There are numerous reasons why such testing might be initiated, ranging from pregnancies complicated by chronic medical conditions, such as diabetes, high blood pressure, clotting disorders, anti-inflammatory diseases like lupus, and pregnancies involving multiple gestation (twins, triplets). In conditions such as these, where assessments such as fetal growth and placental function are of considerable concern, NST and BPP testing is typically implemented in the third trimester, sometimes as often as twice weekly.

Non-stress testing, as well as biophysical profiles, are implemented when expectant moms have concerns about general things such as baby not moving as much as usual or meeting kick count criteria, and when pregnancies go beyond their due dates.

The non-stress test is easy to perform. It's our way of assessing fetal heart tones and looking at uterine activity. This is accomplished by connecting two belts around the gravid uterus and looking at the aforementioned. It usually lasts for 20 minutes (at least).

Okay. So, you are sitting in an exam room with these straps connected to you. Just what are we looking for? I get asked this ALL the time. I LOVE when I see my patients watching these two lines, their tracings, dancing along the paper. What does it all mean and exactly what can we interpret from these tracings? The non-stress test is a good indicator of how baby's heart rate responds to fetal movement and can be indicative of problems such as hypoxia, or low oxygen supply. The NST lasts for at least 20 minutes. I say that because if the criteria aren't met, we may leave you on for an extended period of time. What is the criteria? I'm looking for an increase in fetal heart rate of 15 beats above baseline (aka an acceleration), lasting for 15 seconds. If these criteria aren't met, the usual next step is to proceed with a biophysical profile.

The biophysical profile is an ultrasound that looks at a few different parameters, including movement, tone, breathing, amniotic fluid level, and fetal heart rate. Each component is given a score of 0 if criteria are not met or 2 if criteria are met.

In my practice, non-stress testing and biophysical profiles are not implemented until the third trimester, usually no earlier than 28 weeks. If the testing is reassuring, the pregnancy is allowed to continue, though in my practice, if a pregnancy reaches 41 weeks gestation and is still undelivered, we typically pick a date for delivery, whether that be by induction of labor or cesarean section. If, however, the pregnancy is remote from delivery, that is, pre-term, and the testing is not reassuring, then discussions are had regarding further treatment and potentially moving towards delivery.

What's so important about third trimester labs?

Whenever I ask my pregnant ladies how far along in their pregnancies they are, I encourage responding in weeks gestation as opposed to a certain number of months. In pregnancy, it is the weeks that serve as milestones.

I remember my own pregnancy and how ELATED I was about the whole miracle that was eventually to be my daughter. My wife's and my daughter. Ahhh! It was so incredibly exciting, and my wife is such a love, but I tried not to let her know all the ways I was worrying my brains out. I mean, I'm an OB/GYN for crying out loud! I recognized everything that could go wrong in a pregnancy, especially considering I was an "older" gal and all. I used the weeks as landmarks. At 24 weeks I allowed myself to breathe just a bit as this is/was the milestone for viability.

At 28 weeks, I allowed myself to breathe a little bit more. While I prayed that things continued to move along smoothly, in the back of my mind I knew that if our little girl was born at that point, she would have a strong chance of survival thanks the care we were receiving from my perinatologist friends. Not to mention the exemplary care Francesca would certainly receive at the nearby level III center with their amazing team of neonatologists, if it came to that. I had, after all, seen all these amazing professionals in action when they cared for a set of twins I once delivered at around 24 weeks, both of whom are now alive and thriving at twelve years of age (OB/GYN success stories are THE BEST!).

At 32 weeks, I thought to myself, we are almost there, just hang on, girlie; but if you do decide to come now, I am feeling even better about your chances. And then we hit 34 weeks.

WHEEEEEEEEEW! Not taking for granted that 34 weeks is, for all intents and purposes, still considered preterm (remember, you are not considered full term until 37 weeks of gestation, and even at this point, you're considered early term). This landmark is so significant because past this point, if one goes into labor, there are no interventions given to stop delivery. There are no recommendations for fetal steroids or fetal lung maturity at this point. It's important because of all the risks typically associated with pre-term deliveries. Prior to 34 weeks, steroids are primarily given to help with fetal lung maturity, decrease the risks of breathing problems, bowel issues such as necrotizing enterocolitis, and brain bleeds, all of which are associated with prematurity. After 34 weeks, no intervention or attempts to delay delivery through tocolysis (medications to help stop the uterus from contracting long enough to get steroids on board) are given as it is thought that babies will do well on their own after this gestational age, 34 weeks. There has recently been the recommendation to consider administering steroids in the late pre-term period, which is defined as the time frame between 34 and 0/7 weeks and 36 and 6/7 weeks, specifically if delivery is imminent (within seven days). Giving steroids during this time frame is thought to assist in decreasing breathing difficulties and extended stays in the neonatal intensive care unit. Both of which are common in babies born prematurely.

Not to minimize all the risks and concerns that are associated with prematurity, but once we hit the 34-week mark, it was pretty much smooth sailing until 36 weeks... when everything came to a SCREECHING HALT!

YOU WANT TO DO WHAT? Remember, I have already told you about the interesting dynamic between myself and the obstetrician that managed my pregnancy. Not only was she one of the partners in my former practice, but she is also my dear friend!

I'm talking about the group B strep test. This test is generally performed around 36 weeks and involves obtaining a culture via a probe that's inserted just inside the vagina, traced down the perineum (the skin between the vagina and the rectum) and, gulp, then a poke inside the rectum.

I know we've already spoken about this, and I can totally admit that I was just as apprehensive about this test as most of you probably are, so, when given the option to do it myself, well, I did just that. They definitely didn't tell me about this perk in med school, ha! It is a running joke between me and this colleague turned friend turned OB. To be honest, I don't really think she thought I, we, actually, would do it. She stepped out of the room for something and when she left I told my wife exactly what to do and she did it. I don't think a rectal swab counts as a date, but I sure did love my lady in that moment. By the time my OB returned to the room we were done. Of course, she stood there in disbelief saying, "Ang, I was just kidding." We in turn replied, "Well, we weren't. Here's your GBS culture. And regarding checking my cervix, I'm not having any problems. No leaking, contractions, or pressure, so that won't be necessary." Granted, it wouldn't have been the first time my doctor saw my girl parts, but I liked to make those occasions as few and far between as possible. I told you I can be old-school!

Some obstetricians start doing routine cervical exams around 36 weeks gestation, but I don't generally follow that rule of thumb. I need a reason to check you. If you are noting contractions, pressure, and leaking of fluid, I'm more inclined to do so, but not just because you are 36 weeks. No need to rock the boat, baby.

We've already discussed another lab test that is typically obtained in the third trimester -- you know, the screening test for gestational diabetes, the one-hour glucola test. Well, along with this one, we also repeat a complete blood count as well as conduct HIV testing.

Regarding the repeat CBC (complete blood count), it is not uncommon to get dilutional anemia during pregnancy. This is often the result of the increased intravascular (blood) volume that is a direct result of pregnancy itself. I always remind my ladies that their intravascular volumes increase by at least 50 percent to maintain and support their current pregnancies. This increase is a cumulative result of the increases that are seen in both plasma volume as well as red blood cell production. The physiological or delusional anemia some women experience in pregnancy are direct results of disproportionate increases in plasma volumes in comparison to red blood cell production.

In most cases, anemia in pregnancy is due to iron deficiency and is typically treated with supplemental iron. However, there are many other causes of anemia, including, sickle cell anemia, vitamin B12 or folate deficiency, underlying chronic medical conditions such as kidney disease, or acute blood loss. So, while it may be common place to experience things such as tiredness and shortness of breath during the course of a normal pregnancy, it's important to have these third trimester labs done to ensure that there is nothing more significant going on.

RhoGAM? What's the big deal?

As we touched on earlier, part of your prenatal battery includes testing your blood type, Rh factor, and antibody screen. You are probably quite familiar with blood types (A, B, AB, O) and the positive or negative often mentioned along with your blood type. Say for instance you are O+ (positive). That positive or negative connotation alludes to whether or not you have tested positive for being a carrier of the Rh antigen, which is a protein marker on your blood. If you are Rh positive, keep on keepin' on, however, if you are Rh negative, which means you are not a carrier of the Rh antigen, then at 28 weeks, or at the time of your third trimester lab draw, you will receive a shot of RhoGam. The reason for this is that if you are Rh negative and baby is Rh positive, and there is any mixing of your bloods (which can occur on such occasions as trauma, amniocentesis, childbirth, miscarriage, or pregnancy termination), sensitization can occur and, as a result, maternal antibodies can form against the baby's Rh antigen.

Why is that a problem? Because this exposure can have serious implications for future pregnancies. To prevent this sensitization or exposure, Rho (D) immunoglobulin, aka, RhoGAM, is given at 28 weeks and at the time of delivery to any mom that is Rh negative. RhoGAM may also be given if there were signs of bleeding during pregnancy, at the time of invasive procedures such as an amniocentesis and CVS (chorionic villus sampling), or if there have been instances of trauma.

CHAPTER 9
HIGH RISK PREGNANCIES

Going into my own pregnancy it was already a given that I would be considered high-risk. My age alone catapulted me into this category. Remember, I was 37 years old when I had Francesca. Also, our pregnancy was a "modern" one of sorts, with two moms, something that isn't always so well-received in the conservative Midwest. While this twist wasn't a medical risk, it certainly proved to be an emotional stressor, at times leaving my wife and I to deal with the perceptions of others who just didn't quite understand how or why two women would have a baby.

What makes a pregnancy high-risk?
When most of us hear the phrase high-risk, all of a sudden, we freak out and think the worst. Even wackier, I have patients that consider the phrase high-risk some kind of badge of honor.

Slow down, Sally! Let's not put the cart before the horse!

The fact of the matter is, I find that most patients either don't truly have high-risk pregnancies and plenty of us don't understand what really makes a pregnancy high-risk. Furthermore, most high-risks pregnancies, aside from being monitored more closely, which, in layman's terms, translates into more frequent visits to your OB/GYN's office and increased antepartum testing, end up doing well and delivering at full term.

So just what does make a pregnancy high-risk? Any pre-existing medical condition that has the potential to adversely affect the pregnancy. Things such as:

Obesity

Chronic hypertension

Extremes in age; teen pregnancy or being advanced maternal age (over the age of 35)

Autoimmune disorders (lupus is an example)

Bleeding or clotting disorders

Pre-existing diabetes

Renal disease

Cardiac disease

Or, any condition that develops during pregnancy that has the potential to adversely affect the pregnancy. For example:

Gestational diabetes

Multiple gestation (twins, triplets, quadruplets)

Preeclampsia

Incompetent cervix

Preterm labor

Placenta previa

Having a pre-existing medical condition like those noted above certainly puts your pregnancy at risk for numerous issues ranging from growth concerns (baby being too large or small) to early delivery (specifically, before 37 weeks). If you either have, or are at risk of, developing a high-risk pregnancy, it simply means that we will be keeping a much closer eye on you and baby. This typically entails implementation of some sort of antepartum testing, which translates into get used to seeing your OB/GYN. A lot.

What is preeclampsia?

While there are tons of medical conditions that can catapult you into high-risk classification, either preexisting or ones that develop during the course of a pregnancy, preeclampsia and gestational diabetes are the two I most commonly encounter. Let's start with preeclampsia. What is it?

Preeclampsia is an entity that can only be diagnosed after the 20th week of pregnancy. Its signifiers are high blood pressure and a certain amount of protein in your urine. If we MUST be technical about it, high blood pressure is diagnosed when you have a systolic blood pressure (the top number) greater than or equal to 140 and/or a diastolic blood pressure (the bottom number) greater than or equal to 90. Got that? Both numbers don't have to be elevated, just one or the other. In preeclampsia, this happens in conjunction with proteinuria, or having a certain amount of protein in your urine, 300 mg obtained by way of a 24-hour urine collection (YES, that bizarre THING where you have to pee in a jug for an entire day and night and then hand it over to the lab). A urine dip of 1+ protein is also diagnostic. These just make up the basis of the diagnosis.

The deal with preeclampsia is that it can affect other organ systems such as kidneys, your GI (gastrointestinal) tract, and neurological systems. If these other systems become involved, the diagnosis goes from basic preeclampsia---and I'm not even sure if there even is such a thing as basic preeclampsia since it's serious regardless) to severe preeclampsia. No bueno!

We are able to diagnose you as being severe via laboratory evaluation or the development of certain symptoms, such as:

Headaches that don't go away with minimal intervention like Tylenol.

Heartburn that won't abate with everyday treatments such as Tums.

RUQ (right upper quadrant) pain that is not relieved with positional changes nor is it gas related.

Visual changes such as blurry vision or seeing spots that are not the result of staring into a bright light.

Abnormal lab work like low platelet counts, elevated liver function tests, abnormal renal tests (especially elevated creatinine).

All these are examples of things that you might experience if you have severe preeclampsia.

The treatment for preeclampsia is delivery, but depending on how far along you are in the pregnancy, this can prove tricky, and the risks and benefits of conservative management versus delivering a pre-term baby have to be weighed.

I hate preeclampsia! Even after all these years, no one really knows what even causes the stupid thing. Most hypothesize that it's placental in origin. Preeclampsia can be a real MOTHER*&%$#! Sometimes random or even atypical in its presentation, at times preeclampsia can be a complicated diagnosis to make. And don't get me started on the magnesium sulfate that is often times thrown onboard as part of treatment to prevent seizures (eclampsia). You won't like the warm and not so fuzzy feeling you get from this additive!

Here's a perfect example. One evening, while on-call, I'm hanging out at home, catching up on all my DVR'd shows, eating a late-night snack, CHILLIN'! My wife and daughter are out of town visiting family, and for once, it's nice to just be all by myself, work phone not ringing, just hanging out. As I may have mentioned, hanging out on-call is a very rare occasion for me, so, out of the blue, my work phone rings.

"This is Dr. Angela."

No answer. Crickets on the other end. Sometimes it freaks patients out when the actual physician answers the phone, so I answered again. "Dr. Angela here."

The patient finally answered. "Dr. Angela, I'm a G3P2002 at 34 weeks and I just don't feel right. I have this midsternal pain that just won't go away and is radiating to my back, I have had nausea and some vomiting that's still going on, and I have a headache and am seeing spots."

Right away in the back of my mind, I'm thinking, HERE WE GO! I immediately send the patient in for evaluation and call labor and delivery, giving them the heads up on this patient's impending arrival. I ask them to obtain some basic lab work on her thinking in the back of my mind that this could be preeclampsia. DAMN, DAMN, DAMN.

I receive a call from the nurse, much too soon I might add, I know that they haven't gotten those labs back yet. The nurse informs me that the first series of blood pressures for this expectant mother are 200s/100s. By blood pressure criteria alone I know that this is likely preeclampsia. A severe case. The blood pressure, in conjunction with the other symptoms of headache, visual changes, sternal pain, said something. And the labs, of course, once they finally came back, confirmed my findings: low platelets, elevated creatinine, 3+ protein. The funny thing is, this same patient had just been ruled out for preeclampsia two weeks prior at a routine prenatal visit. She informed me that she had had an episode of high blood pressure and that her laboratory evaluation was within normal limits.

As fate would have it, I had never met this patient before, which is one of the reasons I always encourage patients to meet everyone in the practice, you never know who will be delivering you or taking care of you once you present to labor and delivery. This patient, I'm sure, had no idea she would be delivering at 34 weeks gestation.

As I reviewed the nervous mom's chart and spoke with her, I immediately identified the obvious risk factors this patient had for preeclampsia. Her previous two deliveries were full term and uncomplicated, the last being about eight years ago. So, let's see, advanced maternal age, almost ten years between deliveries, and then it hit me! There was a DIFFERENT FATHER FOR THIS BABY! That was likely the most significant of her risk factors.

She was admitted, started on magnesium sulfate, given medications to control her blood pressure, and delivered. Talk about crazy! There is no rhyme or reason to preeclampsia and it often is diagnosed either at a routine office visit or randomly, as was the case with this patient.

Risk factors include being a first-time mom, extremes in age (teen or advanced maternal age), any of the autoimmune disorders (like lupus), diabetes, multiple gestations (twins, triplets), obesity, renal disease, previously affected pregnancy, or different paternity from previous children, just to name a few.

That said, puh-lease don't panic, there is an entire arsenal of treatment options to combat this monster! Whether it's controlling elevated blood pressure with various medications or initiating all sorts of antepartum testing to ensure that you and baby are okay, we've got you covered!

Why does gestational diabetes make me high-risk?

I used to always say, "If God TRULY EVER wants to get back at me, He would make me a gestational diabetic." I mean, who can take checking your blood sugars via finger prick four times a day? Not this weeny! I mean, sure, we ultimately do what we have to do, but that in and of itself is, like, a death sentence to me. This message was brought to you by THE WORLD'S BIGGEST CHICKEN!

Let's start with the diagnosis of gestational diabetes, the one-hour glucola. Between 26 and 28 weeks, you will be subjected to the one-hour glucola, the official screening test for gestational diabetes. This is not a fasting test. You will be required to drink a 50-gram sugary drink flavored in lemon-lime, cola, or orange. I don't think it matters much which flavor you opt for, or even whether you consume this beverage hot or cold. They all kind of suck. I HATED the taste. Like drinking super sweet, flat, soda. Blech!

An hour after consumption, your blood will be drawn, and your sugar levels tested. Depending on which scale your OB uses, a number below 130 or 140 is usually deemed normal. If, however, you fail the screening test, you will be sent for a diagnostic test, the three-hour glucose tolerance test. Unlike the one-hour glucola, this test does involve fasting. You will not be permitted to consume any food or drink after midnight the evening prior to your scheduled testing. Your blood levels will be drawn upon arrival to the lab (your fasting value), and at one, two, and three-hour intervals. If at least two of the values are abnormal, well, come on down because you have gestational diabetes!

I joke to lighten the mood, but I know this test always has my prego moms on edge. After they take the test the office phones blow up with expectant moms wanting to know their results, like, yesterday. "Do I have it?" They ask and ask and ask. When I do have the test results, they are typically the first things I go over at the next visits. Otherwise, I may as well be speaking Charlie Brown (wa-wa wa, wa-wa, wa), as nothing I say will stick due to my moms-to-be wondering whether or not they have to take the three-hour glucola or not.

If I have a patient with risk factors for gestational diabetes---non-Caucasian, over the age of 25, overweight, family history of diabetes, previously affected pregnancy, or previous macrosomic (large baby) child at birth---I will order an early glucola test. Not only will I have an early screening test done, but I will repeat it between 26 and 28 weeks.

Not to fear. A gestational diabetes diagnosis does not mean that you will automatically be on insulin. The next step usually involves meeting with a diabetic educator who will review dietary modifications and how to measure your blood sugars. Remember, this is four times a day and includes a fasting value as well as two-hour postprandial values. Translation: two hours of testing after breakfast, lunch, and dinner. The hope is that you'll be able to control your blood sugars with diet and exercise alone. If not, we usually initiate you on some sort of insulin, whether that be in pill or injectable forms. If you do happen to be diagnosed with gestational diabetes and your blood sugars are well controlled and managed without insulin, we typically manage your pregnancy just as any other pregnancy. If, however, you require insulin, you can expect to see a lot more of us as you will undergo increased fetal surveillance. This usually includes non-stress tests, biophysical profiles, and growth ultrasounds. In my practice, we see insulin-requiring diabetics twice weekly and they usually have growth ultrasounds every three to four weeks.

The timing of delivery is typically dependent on the results of the testing.

I know, being diagnosed with gestational diabetes is no fun at all. I totally get it. Between the finger sticks four times a day (ouch!), the increased office visits (hello, you have a life), and that fetal surveillance, which can seem to take forever, the whole experience might drive you totally insane. Remember, above all, our objective here is to ensure that you have a good outcome, which means giving birth to a healthy baby. Any sort of fetal surveillance is done to safeguard just that, as poorly controlled diabetes certainly does increase the risk for fetal loss.

Gestational diabetes definitely puts you at an increased risk for hypertensive disorders such as preeclampsia as well as things like pre-term labor. With pre-term delivery and diabetes (not a good combination), the baby will certainly be at an increased risk for respiratory issues. We are always concerned with the sizes of babies born to moms affected with gestational diabetes as all the extra sugar in mom's bloodstream can lead to an increase in insulin production by the baby's pancreas, which in turn can lead to a BIG baby. The size of the baby can potentially alter the route of delivery and lead to things such as shoulder dystocia or labor abnormalities. Babies of diabetic mothers are also at an increased risk for electrolyte abnormalities as well as low blood sugar after delivery. These things are monitored very closely.

Having gestational diabetes also puts both you and baby at an increased risk for developing diabetes later in life. Obesity is also a major concern, which leads me to stress the importance of diet and exercise. Lifestyle alterations can have major impacts on health in general. Not just during pregnancy, but post-delivery as well.

Mothers affected by gestational diabetes typically undergo additional screening tests six to 12 weeks post-delivery to ensure that the diabetes has resolved. Usually this is done with a 75-gram oral glucose tolerance test. If this test is normal, moms are usually screened every three years or so due to the increased risk of developing diabetes later on in life.

Gestational diabetes is quite common in pregnancy. Though I am grateful to have not been affected by it during my own pregnancy, I take care of plenty of moms who are. Through concerted efforts between the pregnant mom, the specialist, and the general OB/GYN, it is a rare occasion that I see any of the complications that can result from poorly controlled gestational diabetes. Most of my moms with gestational diabetes, both those who are diet and insulin controlled, end up with healthy, happy babies.

CHAPTER 10
SIGNS AND SYMPTOMS OF LABOR

It all comes down to this. The main event. Labor. Let me tell you, they don't call it that for nothing. Labor is work. All of the aches and pains, moans and groans, sleepless nights -- everything is leading up to the imminent birth of your bundle of joy! Roll out the red carpet because it's time for the show.

Is losing my mucus plug the same thing as going into labor?
No, ma'am, it's not!
I can't begin to tell you how many panicked phone calls I get during the wee hours of the morning or final hours of the day with declarations of, "Dr. Angela, I just lost my mucus plug! Now what?"
This totally cracks me up because when one does lose her mucus plug, well, I hate to be a Debbie Downer but there are no fireworks that miraculously illuminate the sky, or confetti that suddenly falls from above. There is no sudden *POP* of champagne corks or Ed McMahon randomly appearing out of nowhere to hand you a million-dollar check.
My usual response to the statement of losing the mucus plug, after having a little smile of my own, is "Are you having any contractions associated with this?" If the answer is no, there is nothing to do except continue what we have been doing. Waiting. I hate to break it to you, but losing your mucus plug isn't as big a deal as it's been made out to be.
So, just what is a mucus plug? Exactly that, a gathering of cervical mucus that guards entry into the uterus. Literally, a plug. I usually tell expectant mamas that losing the mucus plug is just a sign that the normal changes that occur in our bodies as we get closer and closer to delivering baby are transpiring. Losing the mucus plug just means that the cervix is getting ready. It's softening, dilating, and thinning out in preparation for the upcoming delivery.

For those of you who don't know what a mucus plug looks like, trust me, I know, and so you don't need to store it in a napkin or plastic bag to bring to the office for me to look at. Nor do I need for you to take pictures with your cell phone. I promise, I believe you, and again, I know what it looks like. But for those of you that aren't sure, you may not be able to discern it from your "normal" physiologic discharge. Discharge in pregnancy does increase as you progress further and further along in weeks gestation. It (your mucus plug) might be clear, thick, tinged with blood, slightly yellowish, or greenish. As with most discharge in pregnancy, my usual rule of thumb is the following: As long as it doesn't smell, burn, or itch, it's probably fine.

How will I know if I'm going into labor?
The best response I've heard regarding the above is as follows: You'll know you are in labor when you don't have time to put on full-face makeup before going to the hospital. I about DIED LAUGHING when I heard this. It's so true, though I must admit I do have a few moms that managed to paint eyes, lips, and cheeks prior to coming to labor and delivery, contractions be damned.

I know it can be frustrating for expectant moms to endure regular uterine contractions, get up in the middle of the night, drive all the way to labor and delivery, only to be told, sorry, not yet, and have to go back home. I get it! I wish there were some way for me to look into my clinical crystal ball and discern true labor versus a false alarm. I always ask my ladies to find solace in the fact that when they have to go in, if I'm on-call, I have to go in, too! Trust me, I'm not thrilled about having to go in for false alarms either but, as they say, it is what it is!

By definition, labor is characterized by uterine contractions that result in cervical change. So, as you have probably figured out by now, you can have uterine contractions without actually being in labor. As a matter of fact, it is not uncommon to have uterine contractions once you enter the third trimester and your uterus prepares for labor and delivery. I usually instruct my patients to time their contractions. While the recommendation of when to call differs from provider to provider, I usually recommend calling for uterine contractions that are seven minutes or less apart and have been present for more than an hour. Another factor to consider is whether or not your water has broken (this isn't always as dramatic as depicted on television or the movies. Sometimes there isn't a big gush or flood; it can be as slight as a continuous trickle). And of course, if any of the usual concerns come up, like baby isn't moving or meeting kick count criteria, or active bleeding, and I'm not talking blood-tinged mucus as noted above. If ever there is any uncertainty, JUST CALL. Remember, this is what your doctor does for a living!

Leading up to these signs and symptoms you may have noticed feeling as if baby is "dropping." I'm a huge fan of measuring fundal heights (you know, when we take that measurement from the pubic symphysis to the top of your uterus, aka your uterine fundus) so I usually mention if I see, based on measurement, that the baby is dropping.

Can't imagine having any more discharge than you've already had during the course of this pregnancy? Well get ready to ride the wave, mama, because you might notice increased discharge at this point. Your obstetrician may also inform you that your cervix is starting to dilate, soften, thin out, and that baby is well-engaged in the pelvis. You may also start experiencing even more lower back and pelvic pain. While these are normal parts of pregnancy thanks to hormones, specifically relaxin, making all your joints and ligaments feel loosey-goosey, these feelings become more exaggerated as one approaches and enters labor. All in preparation for the delivery of baby.

Other not so fun things you might notice include diarrhea (it's not just the joints and ligaments that loosen up) and feeling DOG TIRED again (and you thought that was just a first trimester thing, pfft).

How do I know if my water breaks?
I know I already said it but it's worth repeating. Most of the time when a woman's water breaks it isn't NEARLY as dramatic as depicted in the movies or on television. It's not like, all of a sudden, the floodgates open or a dam is suddenly released, and all this fluid just starts pouring out of you. It may be a gush of fluid or a thin, continuous trickle. Honestly, sometimes it's hard to discern whether or not it's your "water" versus just flat out peeing in your pants, which, as we all know, does happen. Just one of the many joys of being pregnant!

My general rule of thumb: IF YOU DON'T KNOW, YOU BETTER ASK SOMEBODY. This rule is applicable across the board, regardless of the inquiry.

Get this: Less than 15 percent of pregnant women actually experience their water breaking. If you think it happened and you're not quite sure, there are a couple of ways to try and discern on your own. If your water has truly broken, it's not just going to break, and then all of a sudden, nothing else comes out. You typically continue to leak fluid. Put on a pad and if you soak it, you can pretty much rest assured that your water probably has really broken. Another trick is to lay on your bed or couch so that you are slightly propped up (remember, it's never good to lie flat on your back) and remain in this position for 20 minutes or so. If your water has truly broken, this maneuver will allow the fluid to pool in your vagina; hence, when you stand up, gravity takes over, and voila, the pooled fluid falls out.

Now, occasionally, if you have a "slow leak," I will have to meet you at the hospital. Sometimes the nurses can just look at you and tell that you're grossly ruptured (that just means your perineum is really wet), other times they perform a test that checks the pH of your fluid via a swab. Based on this, we can also usually tell if you're really ruptured. If, however, these maneuvers fail, I usually do a sterile speculum exam. "Everyone's FAVORITE exam!" said no one ever. During this procedure I visualize the cervix and look for fluid pooled in the vagina. If I see it, I usually check the pH and analyze it under a microscope for characteristic findings, a process called ferning because, upon drying and crystallizing, amniotic fluid actually does look like a fern. Kind of gross and kind of beautiful all at the same time (now that's a slogan for pregnancy if I've ever heard one). If I don't see any fluid in the vault, I may also have you cough to see if any fluid leaks from your cervix.

There are other, more involved, techniques that can be utilized to rule in or out rupture of membranes, but I would prefer not to go into these as I very rarely use them. Last but not least, we can always do an ultrasound to see what the amniotic fluid level is. If there is low fluid, and the story is convincing, that's pretty much a sure sign that your water has broken.

My six-year-old daughter, Francesca, is absolutely fascinated with certain aspects of what I do. She gets very excited when I tell her about the babies I have delivered, almost as excited as me! Needless to say, once you have children, you realize that they see and hear EVERYTHING! I swear, I'm sure that between her and my wife, they could triage most of my patients. One evening my work phone rings. The resident on the other end tells me that a woman is in active labor and wants an epidural. I tell him to get her admitted, get her prepped for the epidural, and I will break her water once she is comfortable. Thinking that my mini-me was sleeping, and yes, she likes to sleep in mommy's bed with mama when I'm on call, she rolls over and asks, "Mommy, when the lady's water breaks, is that like her peeing on herself?" I couldn't stop grinning -- proud mom, proud OB/GYN. Pondering how to break this down for my then six-year-old, I think about how my wife and I keep it pretty 100---as in percent---real. I say to my lovebug, "Remember how mommy told you that babies swim in a bag of fluid inside the mother's uterus, where baby lives inside of mommy? Well, sometimes if that bag breaks, either on its own or if mommy bursts it, all the fluid comes out. While it may look like the mom is peeing on herself, it's not pee, just the fluid that baby was swimming in." And to that, she responds, "Okay," and rolls over and goes to sleep.

You'll know it soon enough: kids are just the best.

What are Braxton Hicks contractions?
Braxton Hicks contractions are your uterus' way of gearing up for the main event: LABOR! As I tell all my pregnant moms, labor means work. In order for us to utilize our muscles to the best of their abilities, we have to train them. Braxton Hicks contractions are your body's way of doing just that, training your uterus for the huge responsibility of pushing the baby out. Braxton Hicks contractions typically commence around 20 weeks of gestation and tend to be infrequent in occurrence, though you may start to experience them more noticeably as you enter into your third trimester of pregnancy. Word to the wise, keep a pulse on these contractions as they can, at times, be difficult to distinguish from real contractions. If you feel as if you are having Braxton Hicks, which can become somewhat uncomfortable, guzzle (and keep guzzling) some water or try moving around and changing positions. If none of these actions help, and the contractions continue to be uncomfortable, please do not hesitate to call your physician. I once took a call from a patient who thought she was having Braxton Hicks, but we subsequently decided it a good idea to have her evaluated on labor and delivery. Boy was I happy that we did. She was truly in labor!

How far apart should contractions be before I call my doctor?
This is totally provider dependent. I typically instruct my patients to call me if their contractions are seven minutes or less apart and have been persistent beyond one hour. Of course, I also tell my patients to call me if they have any questions, issues, or concerns. The thought of baby finally arriving can be enough to make one lose all mental function and ability to properly assess all that is presently happening. When this occurs I typically get fathers-to-be making the calls for their wives or partners, which is a complete nightmare because, most of the time, these guys haven't been to many or any of the prenatal visits and can't tell me how many weeks pregnant their ladies are, let alone tell me about whether or not labor is occurring. So once I've gotten the true patient on the phone, I'm able to take a history, discern what is going on, and give proper instructions, which can be I don't think this is labor, no need to come in, or, this is it, I'll see you at the hospital!

CHAPTER 11
DELIVERY TIME

How will I know if I need a C-section?

Your OB/GYN will tell you.

I always encourage my expectant moms to be sure they take active roles in their care, whether it's the antepartum visits or during labor and delivery. Ask a lot of questions! Remember, this is your experience. YOU should be aware and a part of most, if not all, decisions pertaining to you and baby! Never forget what GI Joe said, "Knowing is half the battle!" So, if you can manage that, you can take on whatever comes next.

Labor and delivery nurses are an AMAZING group that not only provide exemplary care but typically serve as the biggest advocates for mothers-in-waiting. They often play liaison between you and your physician, especially if you are shy or reluctant to speak up.

If things aren't moving in the right direction, whether labor has stalled in spite of last-ditch efforts to jumpstart things or there is a non-reassuring fetal heart tracing, both your nurse and OB/GYN should convey these things to you. I try to let my patients know things step-by-step. I express any concerns I might have, and why I/we may be implementing certain maneuvers or plans. That way, if we do end up in a C-section, due to fetal intolerance to labor, an arrest disorder of some sort (whether it be an arrest of dilation or descent), a maternal indication such as exhaustion (mom being too tired to continue with efforts to push baby out), or whatever the reason may be, communication is key. No matter how sticky the situation may be, I always keep the lines between my team and patients wide open. You deserve to understand what's going on with your body and chime in on how to handle it.

All that good stuff said, there certainly are instances where an emergency C-section must be performed. There are numerous reasons why this may be necessary with a few indications being a uterine rupture, umbilical cord prolapse, and NRFHTs (non-reassuring fetal heart tones) with failure to return to a normal pattern.

When would I need a C-section?

While there are times when we won't be able to predict whether or not a C-section will be needed, there are plenty of occasions where we know well ahead of time that a C-section will occur:

Scheduled Repeat C-sections: You've already had a C-section, for whatever reason, and have opted for another. You have, in essence, refused TOLAC (trial of labor after a C-section) and VBAC (vaginal birth after a C-section). Scheduled repeats are typically performed at 39 weeks gestation (if you don't go into labor prior to then).

Malpresentation: Baby isn't facing the right way, head down.

Multiple Gestation: Twins, when the presenting twin isn't head down, or a higher multiple pregnancy such as triplets or quads.

Placental Issues: Ever heard of a placenta previa? This condition occurs when the placenta either completely or partially covers the cervix. You cannot deliver vaginally with this condition.

Suspected Fetal Macrosomia: We think your baby is too big to fit through your birth canal, whether it be due to baby just being large or you having an inadequate pelvis. If upon having an ultrasound your estimated fetal weight is 5,000g (for non-diabetics), or 4,500g (for diabetics whether pre-existing or gestational), you may be offered an elective C-section by your OB/GYN.

Infections: Certain infections, such as HIV and HSV, may require you to have a C-section. You may or may not be able to have a vaginal delivery with HIV depending on your viral load, and if you have an active herpes outbreak, you will most certainly need a C-section.

Maternal Indication: Sometimes expectant moms have chronic medical conditions that preclude them from delivering vaginally. Certain forms of heart disease where the stress of labor could ultimately prove to be too much for the mother are examples of this.

You may also have a C-section if you have a recently diagnosed pregnancy condition such as preeclampsia or if delivery is indicated yet you are remote from delivery and the condition is either worsening or no progression with current induction of labor is noted. Other scenarios may be that antepartum fetal testing has dictated delivery of baby due to something like IUGR (intrauterine growth restriction) or oligohydraminios (low fluid) and baby is not tolerating labor, or biophysical profile testing is such that immediate delivery of baby is warranted.

Do I need a birth plan?
Remember, THIS IS ALL ABOUT YOU. If you feel you need a birth plan, have a birth plan.
Now, just what exactly is a birth plan?
A birth plan is whatever you want it to be -- there are no rules. Your birth plan sums up what your expectations are during your labor and delivery process. Remember, this is a process. Also, please keep in mind that what you expect isn't always what actually happens. Labor is, to say the least, quite unpredictable.
What little nuggets of information may you have in your birth plan, you ask? Try these on for size:
How many people you want in the room while giving birth.
What you expect for pain management (epidural versus no epidural; IV pain meds versus going au natural).
Whether or not you want continuous or intermittent monitoring.
Delayed cord cutting or immediate cord clamping and cutting.
Immediately putting baby to breast versus getting baby cleaned up prior to being given to mom.
Some moms will request certain music be played, laboring in certain positions, some will want to limit the number of vaginal exams. As you can see, you've got the green light to include just about anything in your birth plan.
Most of my patients don't have birth plans, instead opting to have integral roles in their prenatal care and be active parts of the decision-making process from conception to delivery. However, if you do decide to have a birth plan, remember to grant yourself some flexibility, as at times birth plans can go right out the window once you are in the throes of labor. As Wendy Williams (shout-out to my Jersey sisters!) always says, "A girl's allowed to change her mind."

How long is labor?
WHAT A LOADED QUESTION! I so wish I had the answer to this, but like so much of pregnancy, and life for that matter, the experience is different for everyone. I often tell patients that if I were able to predict how long labor would be for each of my pregnant moms, I would no longer be in the practice of medicine. I would have hit the lottery ten times over and be off lounging in some far-off tropical land. With umbrella-adorned drinks. And endless sun.
No, seriously, that's how unpredictable labor is. If I could figure it out I would be TIME's Woman of the Year.
First off, let me start by saying that labor isn't just labor, it's actually comprised of three stages. Yes, you read that correctly. There are indeed

three stages of labor! Now, don't panic, take a deep breath, and let's go through this.

STAGE ONE:

During this stage, you will start to have regular uterine contractions that will begin to affect cervical change. This is typically referred to as latent labor or early labor. You will notice that you are starting to breathe more through your contractions, you may have to take a pause between routine activities like walking, and you may start to feel more pressure in your pelvis. My recommendation is to call your OB/GYN when your contractions are seven minutes or less apart and more than an hour has passed and you're still having them.

While this is usually enough to send my first-time moms straight to labor and delivery, my moms who have been through this before, recognizing the feeling as early labor, may tend to hold off on calling the on-call OB or presenting to the hospital as they prefer to do some of the laboring at home. Some things that may help to relieve pain and discomfort during this early stage of labor include taking a warm shower or bath, walking, increasing your water intake, having your partner or spouse give you a massage, and practicing your breathing techniques.

Early labor can last up to 12 hours for newbie moms but tends to be shorter with subsequent deliveries. We don't consider you to be in active labor until your cervix has reached about 5cm dilation.

In the active phase of labor, your cervix will dilate at a much more rapid pace. For some of you, it probably felt as if you were going to be in early labor FOREVER! Active labor lasts until you are completely dilated, that is, your cervix is 10cm.

Active labor, just like it sounds, is where all the action takes place. Upon entering into active labor, you will start feeling more frequent and intense contractions (and you thought it couldn't get any worse). Your water may or may not break on its own. You'll start feeling more pressure and some women will experience nausea and even vomiting as the body prepares for the upcoming delivery. You may even experience what I call the pre-delivery shakes. For those of you who opted not to get the epidural for pain relief, positional changes, breathing techniques, and cool compresses to your forehead may help you get more comfortable. Please don't worry about those bodily functions (possibly pooping). While it doesn't happen to everyone, it's a very normal part of the process. I promise that you won't lose any cool points if it happens to you. In fact, as soon as baby arrives no one will remember it or any of the crazy obscenities you may have been hurling at your doctor, partner, nurse, or family, during this insane and amazing process. Let me tell you, pregnant women are some of the most creative cursers I've ever met.

STAGE TWO:

The second stage of labor happens once you are completely dilated, ending with the birth of bouncing baby. It can last anywhere from a few minutes to a few hours, depending on maternal pushing efforts, whether or not it is your first baby (it typically goes faster with subsequent deliveries), and if you've had an epidural, which can sometimes affect pushing efforts as moms may not be able to actually feel the urge to push or tell exactly where to push. If the latter is the case, the epidural can either be turned off or decreased.

So, you're completely dilated, now what?

Well, I trained with a bunch of midwives and prefer to take a hands-off approach. I like to let your body and baby do most of the work and tell me when it's time. Ever heard of the phrase "laboring down?" Well, that's just what I previously described. Once you are completely dilated, we let baby descend into the pelvis and the pushing begins once you have the urge to do so. Pushing too soon can lead to you, the mom, getting tired, as well as cervical swelling. The other reason I like to let moms labor down is that it allows for babies to gradually stretch the perineum (the skin between your vaginal opening and your rectum). This, I find, helps decrease the occurrence of lacerations.

My biggest piece of advice during pushing is to PUSH LIKE YOU'RE HAVING THE BIGGEST BOWEL MOVEMENT OF YOUR LIFE! Those are the muscles you need to use. Also, try to focus on something in the room, whether it be your spouse/partner, a spot in front of you, whatever works. This will prevent you from closing your eyes and keeping the energy of the push in your face. Trust me, you don't want to blow your top.

STAGE THREE:

Remember in The Wizard of Oz when the Wizard tells Dorothy and her crew to "pay no attention to the man over there," as they had just discovered he was hiding behind the curtain pushing all sorts of buttons and controls? Well, I'm going to tell you to do the same thing. Your focus at this point should be on meeting and greeting your brand-new baby boy or girl. At this stage, my focus is on delivering your placenta. This may take anywhere from a few minutes to 30 minutes. Delivery of the placenta will involve your OB/GYN manually massaging your uterine fundus (the top of your uterus) to encourage separation while, at the same time, providing gentle, downward cord traction on the placental/umbilical cord.

After the placenta has been delivered, it will be inspected to ensure that it is intact and complete, (as retained placenta can be a source of postpartum bleeding) and has a three-vessel cord. Your vagina, cervix, and perineum will also be inspected to ensure that there are no lacerations requiring repair.

Will an epidural slow down my labor?

This is a very common misconception. No. The epidural will NOT slow down your labor.

When can I get an epidural?

WHENEVER THE HECK YOU WANT. Long gone are the days when physicians required you to be a certain number of centimeters dilated or in active labor. Some physicians still practice this way, but that's very old-school, even for this old-schooler! Some patients will want an epidural right away due to fear of labor pain, while others tend to take a wait and see approach.

Labor, by definition, means work. You are going to have to put some work in to get this baby delivered. Remember, you are the CEO of this experience. It's all about what YOU want. Getting an epidural doesn't make you any less of a woman and you don't lose any tough chick street cred with me or anyone else for that matter. You already have my utmost respect for even opting to go through labor. Remember, I had an elective C-section because I was/am the biggest chicken imaginable. Even getting the IV was traumatizing for me!

Because labor and delivery is a busy place, I usually recommend you get an epidural sooner than later, especially considering there are a number of things that have to happen once you decide to get the injection. For starters, us docs have to aggressively hydrate you via IV. This helps counteract some of the potential consequences of the epidural, like low blood pressure and negative effects on fetal heart rate. Then we have to make sure the anesthesiologist is available. Remember, while this process is all about you, the anesthesiologist is a pretty popular guy or gal and their presence is requested from here to Timbuktu. Whether it be in other rooms of the hospital for patients requesting pain medications or in the main OR, these smart cookies get around, and plenty of times hospitals don't have an anesthesia team designated for labor and delivery.

Nobody likes to wait in line---especially when there's a human trying to escape from your vagina! --- and receiving the epidural is typically first come, first served. Hence my recommendation of the sooner the better.

When is the latest I can get an epidural?

Generally speaking, there is no last call for the epidural. As long as you are able to sit still for placement, you can have an epidural. I have had patients who were completely dilated get an epidural because, as we all know, most of the time babies don't just fall out. Even though a mom is completely dilated, there can still be hours of pushing ahead.

Is it true that once you have a C-section you must have a C-section with subsequent pregnancies?

Totally not true, dependent upon the type of incision that was made on your uterus at the time of the original cesarean section. The most commonly used uterine incision is a low transverse incision. If you don't have this type of incision, the VBAC (vaginal birth after cesarean) conversation stops here. Not every woman keeps a memo of what kind of uterine incision she received, so fear not if you are unsure. You can always get this information from your operative report.

The decision to attempt a trial of labor after a C-section (TOLAC) or a vaginal birth after a C-section (VBAC) is one that has to be carefully considered by the individual and her provider. In a nutshell, this has to do with whether or not your physician practices at a hospital that allows VBACs. Is there staff available (anesthesia, another physician, etc.) in case of an emergency? Are you even a good candidate for a TOLAC?

Who does make a good candidate? Well, there are a lot of variables at play. First off, the associated risks and likelihood of success have to be within reason for both you and your physician. For those who attempt a TOLAC, and are deemed a good candidate, the likelihood of having a successful VBAC is around 70 to 80 percent. The risk of uterine rupture, which is, by far, the most significant risk with a TOLAC, is less than one percent. Try getting those odds in Vegas!

Discussing the reason for the initial C-section becomes important, as that may be somewhat predictive of the likelihood of success for an attempted vaginal delivery after a C-section. Attempting a TOLAC when the indication for the original C-section was for a non-recurring indication (such as a breech presentation or multiple gestation) is likely to result in a higher success rate than someone who's original C-section was for an arrest disorder (the cervix wouldn't dilate beyond a certain point or the infant wouldn't descend any further into the pelvis).

Other factors that bode in your favor when contemplating a VBAC include whether or not your current pregnancy has been without issue, you go into spontaneous labor before or by your due date, or you've only had one previous C-section. Certainly, if you've had a previous vaginal delivery that greatly increases your chances for success. Alternatively, factors such as advanced maternal age, gestational age greater than 40 weeks, maternal obesity, and suspicion of a large baby are just a few factors that decrease the likelihood of a successful vaginal delivery after a C-section.

After careful consideration of everything, including the items mentioned above, a woman and her physician can best determine if a TOLAC or VBAC is the right option for her.

The benefits of even considering a VBAC are certainly worth mentioning. They include shorter recovery time, less risk associated with a vaginal delivery versus a C-section, more immediate initiation of mother-baby bonding (though the recent introduction of gentle C-sections may offset this a bit), and certainly future family planning, as repeated C-sections not only become more difficult but also carry increased risks.

What is induction of labor?

Let's start by defining labor. Labor is uterine contractions that bring about cervical change. An induction of labor is an artificial means, whether that be mechanical (more to come on this) or via medication, that causes uterine contractions that lead to cervical change.

I'm sure that we all know of someone who has had an induction. My patients run the gamut from those who are fearful and want no part of it to those who can't wait to schedule their induction because they are tired of being pregnant or want to be home for the holidays or have especially hectic lifestyles.

There are numerous indications for being induced, including:

Being post-term. In my practice, if you've gotten to 41 weeks gestation and haven't delivered, we generally pick a date to induce you. We NEVER allow you to get to two weeks beyond your due date as the risks of remaining pregnant at this point (increased risk of having a large baby, baby having a bowel movement in utero and swallowing it, which can lead to infection or breathing issues, placental malfunction) far outweigh the risks that come with getting you delivered

Fetal indications such as IUGR (intrauterine growth restriction; baby not growing at the expected rate).

Uterine infection.

Spontaneous rupture of membranes without ensuing labor. This is when your water breaks and then nothing happens.

Medical indications such as preeclampsia and diabetes.

Oligohydramnios (low fluid around the baby).

Keep in mind, this list is by no means all-inclusive, but it does touch on some of the more common reasons ladies are induced.

Oh, let's not forget one of the most common indications: elective inductions! Word to the wise, the American College of Obstetricians and Gynecologists has basically FORBIDDEN any elective inductions, inductions that are done for non-medical reasons, prior to 39 weeks of gestation. Not to mention, I always remind patients that induction is not without risks, such as a uterine rupture, and if your cervix is not favorable you are at an increased risk of C-section.

How do you induce labor?

Induction of labor can be accomplished by a number of means, but we'll start with a patient I recently saw. She was over 40 weeks pregnant and after several hours of observation at her hospital and not having made any cervical change, it was determined that she was not yet in labor. She came to my office "tired of being pregnant" and to have an ultrasound to ensure that there was an adequate amount of fluid around baby (here's that antepartum testing I talked about that happens once you go beyond your due date). Anyway, her cervical exam for me was unchanged. We opted to STRIP HER MEMBRANES in order to cause the release of a chemical called prostaglandins, which leads to uterine contractions and, hopefully, labor.

Stripping membranes is an aggressive cervical check where your provider separates the membranes of your amniotic sac from your lower uterine segment. Doctor's note: It is not uncommon to have a little spotting after this procedure has been done. I also do not perform this procedure on patients that are GBS (group B strep) positive. I like to err on the side of caution and don't want to risk spontaneous rupture of membranes or risk a patient going into labor and not having an adequate amount of antibiotics available for treatment.

As previously mentioned, once you reach 41 weeks gestation it is my general practice to pick a date to induce you. Remember our conversation of not letting you go two weeks beyond your due date due to increased risks? Yeah, I never forget it.

At my office, we generally perform a cervical exam. Then, if it is deemed, based on your cervical exam, that your cervix is not what we call "favorable" (ain't that a shady euphemism if I've ever heard one), we will recommend cervical ripening. When speaking of cervixes' favorability, many factors are taken into consideration such as cervical position, has your cervix rotated around from its posterior position to either mid-position or an anterior location, and how thinned out (or effaced) your cervix is. When doctors are considering all of this, patients will often hear the results of their cervical exam: your cervix is 2cm dilated, 50 percent effaced, -3 station.

What station is baby? This has to do with baby's descent into the pelvis in relation to your ischial spines. What is the consistency of your cervix? Is it firm or is it softening up? All these factors are important, as when we induce you, we want to ensure that you have the best possible chance of ending up with a vaginal delivery.

If your cervix is not what we deem to be favorable, a common means of making it more favorable is using a medication called Cervidil. This is a prostaglandin. It looks like a tadpole or anemic tampon (ha!). It is generally placed in the posterior aspect of your vagina, underneath your cervix. It stays in place for 12 hours and its aim is to make your cervix more favorable, that is, softer, more dilated, thinner, and in a more anterior, mid-position. Sometimes Cervidil can even put women into labor! If this isn't your fate, 12 hours after placement, it is removed, and your cervix is re-evaluated. If your cervix still isn't favorable, one option is to either place another Cervidil or move to yet another mode of induction and ripening. Cytotec. This medication, also known as Misoprostol, is another prostaglandin that is used to induce labor and make cervixes more favorable (it sounds like they're vying for Miss Congeniality, right?). We use this medication in an off-label role in the world of obstetrics and gynecology as it is typically used to treat and prevent stomach ulcers. This medication is usually placed in the posterior of the vagina in hopes of either making the cervix more favorable or actually inducing labor. You can also take this medication orally to accomplish the same goal.

Mechanical dilation, or the foley bulb balloon, is probably the least favorite mode of induction and cervical ripening. Who wants a balloon placed into what is sure to be a tight space (your cervix), and then blown up, usually with sterile water or saline? Not this wimp over here! The foley bulb works by causing the cervix to release prostaglandins, which hopefully softens the cervix, causes it to dilate, and thin out. All this in an attempt to either induce labor or make your cervix more "favorable" for induction.

Once your cervix is favorable, we generally administer a medication called Pitocin to initiate uterine contractions that will, hopefully, lead to cervical change. Occasionally, if you've spontaneously gone into labor on your own and stopped contracting or it was determined that your contractions were not strong enough to cause cervical change, Pitocin will be given to augment your labor and make your contractions more regular and stronger. Physicians like to act conservatively, and I'm very much of the belief that less is more. I prefer to induce only for medical indications, so I can allow nature to take its course. I mean, women have been having babies for centuries without all the marvels of modern medicine. While I'm not anti-induction, there's nothing worse than having a woman go through a days-long induction all because her body wasn't ready. And while sometimes prolonged inductions happen just because and in spite of, once again, inductions are NOT without risks. They can put you at an increased risk of C-section as well as an increased risk of postpartum hemorrhage (bleeding).

What are natural ways to induce labor?

We've all heard them before: walking, drinking castor oil (OMG, I CAN'T EVEN IMAGINE!), and having sex. I'm sure we've also heard of the various herbs and home remedies. I think I recall one of my patients telling me that eating lots of pineapple would induce labor. While some of these ideas sound good (eating pineapple) and fun (having sex), there is no data supporting that any of these suggestions work one way or the other.

Not true for nipple stimulation, however. This one actually does induce uterine contractions. Let's get those thumbs and index fingers working, ladies!

How many people can I have in the room during delivery?

This is based on hospital policies and also depends on the rules and regulations of your respective labor and delivery floors. Being the extremely private person that I am, I didn't want any more folks in the room than were necessary. The essential team was there as well as my wife. That. Was. It. I know that everyone says you forget everything in the throes of labor and that you won't care about anyone seeing your girl parts but well, I sure did! I wanted as little exposure as possible.

I have many patients who have an entire entourage present at their delivery. To each her own. My rule is simple: As long as your people don't interfere or get in the way of my people (specifically, my team of nurses and staff for the baby) and don't get near my table and instruments, we're all good. If it's good for you, it's good for me. Remember, this is your experience!

Do you routinely cut episiotomies?

HELL TO THE NO! I say this with such brash enthusiasm because I am continually amazed at the number of physicians that still do routinely cut episiotomies. I will tell you like I tell my patients, cutting routine episiotomies is SO OLD-SCHOOL! And I know I've been ranting and raving about how old-school I am, but this one is just too antiquated for me. Now that's not to say that there aren't occasions when episiotomies are absolutely warranted. If there is an emergency and delivery has to be expedited for either maternal or fetal indications or in cases such as shoulder dystocia, where more room is needed to deliver baby, I will perform an episiotomy.

Who is going to deliver my baby?

There are many ways to answer this question, but, for the most part, it depends on who is on-call when baby decides to enter the world. If you are a scheduled delivery (whether C-section or induction) you will have a much better shot at knowing who will be present during your delivery. But even with inductions, which can sometimes take a bit longer than anticipated, things are definitely subject to change. My advice is that you meet all the physicians and practitioners in your OB's office. That way, there isn't a total stranger looking up from between your legs when it's show time!

Anything else I should know about having a primary elective C-section?

Yeah, I did it. And no matter how crazy insane it sounds, I am a board-certified OB/GYN who opted to have an elective primary cesarean section. I was motivated by that which should not be anyone's driving force: FEAR! I WAS AFRAID OF DELIVERING VAGINALLY! There. I said it. I have seen babies pass through vaginas THOUSANDS of times, way more than enough to know that it was not for me. I don't even care about the occasional loss of bodily functions. I have done many things in my lifetime, but delivering vaginally wasn't going to be one of them and, you know what? I was okay with that.

I have already told you that I am the biggest chicken around! Just ask my wife. Despite my training, I was not the most compliant pregnant patient you ever encountered. Not by a long shot. If I hadn't worked in my own OB/GYN's office (remember, my physician was my partner and friend), I probably wouldn't have made it to most of my prenatal appointments. Well, maybe that's a little extreme. Let's just say that if we hadn't had a lab in the office, I probably wouldn't have gotten any of my labs done or even completed that dreadful screening test for gestational diabetes. I HATE needles, which is probably why I ended up getting stuck 15 times before my IV was initiated for my C-section. As if that wasn't bad enough, they had to replace it in the OR. GEEZ!

Now, don't be fooled. Though I have just said to you that I was afraid of delivering vaginally, I also happen to know just about everything there is to know about deliveries, vaginal and cesarean. That's where my board certification and YEARS of experience come in. When I was pregnant, I knew the risks, benefits, pros, and cons of all my options. I was familiar with what complications might arise and what recovery would look like. I wasn't concerned about pelvic pain, prolapse, urinary stress, or incontinence because most of these things are similar regardless of route of delivery. I knew what I was signing up for when I opted to go with the elective primary cesarean section. I knew that THIS was going to be IT; I knew that my wife and I weren't planning to have any other children. This is significant as risks associated with C-sections increase the more you have. Previa, accreta, increta, procreta, hysterectomy... NONE of these things sound very nice because they aren't. The latter, sadly, too many women know all too well. The former are all placental attachment disorders, which increase with subsequent C-sections and certainly can result in a hysterectomy. YIKES!

Warning: Don't have a C-section based on a third trimester estimated fetal weight obtained by ultrasound! I see this all the dang time. Pregnant moms freaking out because the ultrasound said baby is going to weigh nine pounds some ounces. PUMP YOUR BRAKES! I typically offer my patients a C-section if they are diabetic and estimated fetal weight is 4,500 grams OR if they are non-diabetic and estimated fetal weight is 5,000 grams. Otherwise, you can undergo a trial of labor. If you start falling off the labor curve and aren't making the sort of changes that are typical of labor, you and your OB/GYN should and will talk.

In all honesty, an estimated fetal weight obtained by ultrasound in the third trimester is no better than my bedside Leopold's maneuvers (you know, where I feel your gravid uterus and palpate to determine baby's position as well as guestimate how much I think baby is going to weigh). Through YEARS of experience I've gotten to be pretty darn good at estimating fetal weight by feel, I guess you could say THE FORCE IS STRONG with me in that way. But, still, it ain't hard science.

I've said all of the above to say this (another throwback, this one from Digital Underground): Doowhutchyalike! Don't let fear be the determining factor. Don't have an elective cesarean section based solely on an ultrasound estimate, which can occasionally be correct but I've also seen them be WAY off. See what I'm saying? Know ALL the facts! Risks, benefits, pros, cons. Ask questions. Got it?

CHAPTER 12
POSTPARTUM

When will I be discharged from the hospital?
This depends on your postpartum course (how you recover after delivery).
However, before we can even speak to postpartum course, we must first
see how you delivered. Vaginal or C-section? As you might imagine, the
recovery from a vaginal delivery is typically less cumbersome and somewhat
shorter than that following a C-section.
Various parameters are taken into consideration prior to discharge,
including stability of vital signs, lab results, pain control, mobility, and your
general state of being. Most facilities will have the new mother fill out a
screening questionnaire for postpartum depression to ensure that you aren't
too overwhelmed by the life changing events that have just occurred.

What is the normal course after a vaginal delivery?
The course following a vaginal delivery is routine. As long as there are no
issues, most moms who deliver vaginally are discharged to home on
postpartum day two, postpartum day zero being the actual day of delivery.
Your attending physician will check on you as long as you are in the
hospital. On postpartum day one, we are primarily concerned with your
labs, specifically your hemoglobin and hematocrit, making sure they are
stable and that there are no obvious signs of anemia, whether that be
demonstrated by your labs, vital signs such as low blood pressure,
tachycardia (fast heart rate), or subjective feelings of extreme
tiredness/weakness. Checking for uterine firmness and position post-
delivery are significant aspects of the postpartum evaluation.
Close attention is paid to the amount of bleeding experienced during the
postpartum course to ensure that there hasn't been or won't be a significant
amount of blood loss. Hence the commonly asked question, "How's your
bleeding?" Post-delivery, most moms will experience bleeding like a heavy
period, which should gradually taper with each passing day. This bleeding,
more commonly termed lochia, may last anywhere from six to eight weeks.

Along with gradually decreasing the further outside of the delivery you get, your body will release a veritable Pantone color wheel, with the blood changing from bright red to dark red to brown to tan to white and, eventually, back to your normal clear discharge. As long as such is the case, and there is no foul odor, everything is progressing as expected.

On postpartum day number two, as long as all is well, and the new baby is ready to be discharged, you will get to go home!

Usual follow-up with your obstetrician is six weeks later, so long as there are no issues that require close follow-up, to address things such as blood pressure monitoring or postpartum depression issues.

Word to the wise. As mentioned above, this postpartum bleeding can last anywhere from six to eight weeks. Just when you think it's gone---boom---it's back. To avoid any unwanted surprises, I always advise my ladies to wear a panty liner.

To breastfeed or not to breastfeed? That is the question.

Most postpartum suites have a lactation consultant who visits new mothers and addresses any questions about breastfeeding whether regarding the actual act itself, latching on, or milk supply.

Breastfeeding is an extremely personal choice. Don't allow yourself to be bullied or made to feel bad if your decision varies from what is encouraged or promoted at your facility.

What is the recovery like following a C-section?

Contrary to popular belief, a C-section is a major surgery.

Recovery from a C-section can be smooth sailing, knowing what to expect is half the battle. The actual day of your C-section is considered post-op day zero. Aside from coming to grips with the fact that you won't actually be the first person to hold your new bundle of joy I didn't find the recovery so difficult.

The journey for me started with the IV. Knowing that we were only going to have one child, not to mention the fact that I was terrified of labor, I decided to have an elective primary C-section. I was healthy and had undergone an unremarkable pregnancy. As is with most surgery, you receive instruction not to consume anything after midnight on the day prior to your scheduled procedure.

We arrived at the hospital at some Godforsaken hour the morning of July 17, 2009. I had only just turned my work pager and phone off the night before. I was one of those moms who worked the entire pregnancy.

My wife, dad, and both moms (no, I don't have lesbian mothers, just a dad who remarried) arrived at the hospital with me in tow. The biggest piece of the whole C-section ordeal for me was getting my IV started. I was stuck, I kid you not, about 15 times before the anesthesiologist FINALLY was able to get a line in. This was more traumatizing than the spinal, I didn't even feel that going in. Soon, the meds from the spinal began to take effect. Talk about weird. For about 45 minutes, I knew firsthand what it must feel like to not be able to move your lower extremities. While lying on the operating table I willed myself to move or lift my legs to no avail.

I found the entire team of nurses, both the OR and pediatric teams, to be amazing. While I work with these folks on a daily basis, it really is something different to be on the other side of the curtain. All I really felt was pushing and pulling, I requested not to hear any of the OR chat that typically occurs among the surgeons. Being that I perform this procedure on a regular basis, I did not want to know where they were at any point during my surgery.

Once the procedure was completed, I was wheeled to recovery with IV running and foley (a flexible tube passed through the urethra and into the bladder to drain urine) in place. Speaking of the foley, it isn't as big a deal as you might think. It is typically inserted once you have received your spinal/epidural, or whatever the anesthesiologist is going to give you for your surgery.

I wasn't too sore afterwards. I started with clear liquids and advanced my diet as tolerated, I cannot quite recall what I had for dinner that evening, but it wasn't hospital food.

Post C-section, as with a vaginal delivery, the nurses will keep a very close eye on your vitals, your uterine position to ensure that it remains firm, as well as checking your pad to ensure you aren't bleeding too much.

As noted above, your attending physician will see you each day that you are in the hospital. For moms who delivered via C-section, most are discharged to home on post-op day three. Some may stay until day four if insurance will cover it or if there are issues with the baby.

Post-op day one is the usual assessment of vital signs and lab work to ensure you are not anemic (this can happen if you are bleeding heavily or lost a significant amount of blood during the section). I still listen to heart and lungs at this point and check for the position of the uterus and its firmness. It's important that the uterus remain firm post-delivery so there are less risks of bleeding. Speaking of uteruses, palpating (feeling) the uterus is also important to check for signs of undue tenderness or pain, which could be signs of infection.

The big reveal of post-op day one is the incision. Up to this point, it has been covered with some sort of dressing which typically is removed on post-op day one. In my role as a physician, I typically allow my patients to remove their dressing in the shower. After all, having a bandage taped to your skin removed the first day post-surgery is no fun at all. OUCH! The incision check is just to make sure there are no signs of trouble such as infection or bleeding.

There will always be inquiries about pain control or lack thereof, how heavy your bleeding is, whether or not you are tolerating a regular diet, if you are passing gas, or if you've started moving around.

The big goal of post-op day one is to start moving around. This is usually accomplished once your Foley catheter is removed. Post-op day two is, ta-da, more of the same! Now that you are settling into your role as a new mom, this is the day that you will start preparing for your big journey home. As previously mentioned, most women are discharged to home on post-op day three as long as there are no issues. On the day of discharge, you should be well on your way to feeling like your old self again. The belly is gone, you are moving around, pain control should be adequate, and of course, your exam findings should be such that there are no reservations about sending you home. A review of medications, activity level, and follow-up are all things that should be addressed prior to your going home.

Most moms are discharged to home post-C-section on some sort of narcotic and anti-inflammatory for pain, usually something like Percocet or Vicodin and Ibuprofen or Motrin. Typically, a stool softener (you already know Colace is my jam) is also provided, and maybe iron if there are concerns about anemia.

Wound care is pretty basic, thankfully. I encourage you to get your sponge, rag, whatever, nice and sloppy, soapy wet. Drip the soapy water over your incision, thoroughly rinsing it, and then patting it dry before leaving it open to air. Keeping your incision dry is, in my opinionated opinion, THE most important part of incisional care. If your incision happens to lie under a large pannus (large fold of skin), you can use something like a pad to help keep it dry, however, the pad needs to be changed frequently to ensure that no moisture is in contact with the incision.

Regarding activity, I encourage my new moms not to lift anything heavier than their babies, at least not until after eight weeks or so. If there are stairs in the home, my usual rule of thumb upon arrival home is to decide where you are going to spend most of your day. Once that decision is made, settle in. Going up and down steps isn't a total no-no; a few trips a day post-C-section are acceptable, just don't get all Rocky Balboa, okay?

Typical follow up after a C-section is one to two weeks post-discharge for an incision check at your OB's office. This visit is followed by the usual six-week checkup, which occurs about four weeks later.

Please know, whether or not you are a vaginal or C-section delivery, if there are any concerns, your physician is always happy to see you!

Another pearl of wisdom I always relay to my patients post- discharge is that the swelling in your extremities gets worse before it gets better. So do not be alarmed if you happen to wake up one day, look down, and find that your legs look like tree trunks! This is the body's way of equilibrating by getting rid of all the fluids that were necessary to maintain your pregnancy (the increase in blood volume, not to mention the IV fluids you received while in the hospital), hence the massive fluid shifts. Propping your legs up when you aren't busy (ha, as a new mom you're probably wondering when the heck that is going to be) and drinking water with lemon in it will help you to diuresis the extra fluid away.

Having just delivered, you are still at risk for clotting post-delivery. The risk significantly decreases come six weeks after delivery.

I also encourage moms to continue on their prenatal vitamins, particularly if they are breastfeeding, because there is nothing but good stuff in them.

What birth control is safe if I'm breastfeeding?

I love this question. Usually, the contraception discussion does not take place until you return for your six-week postpartum visit. The six-week time frame is significant, as you remain at an increased risk of clotting until you are at least six weeks post-delivery because of pregnancy hormones. We also wait six weeks to initiate contraception, not only because of the increased risk of clotting prior to this but also to allow an adequate amount of time for the milk supply to be established. Honestly, you could either go on a combination form of contraception (one containing both estrogen and progesterone) or an exclusively progesterone form because there may be a slight decrease in milk supply associated with combination birth control pills -- the operative word here being may. Many women choose to forego taking any chances and go with a progesterone only form of contraception, whether this be a progesterone birth control pill, Depo-Provera, or a progesterone-containing intrauterine device.

Other options for contraception post-delivery include the NuvaRing, a bilateral tubal ligation, and other forms of non-hormonal contraception such as the diaphragm (yes, your mother's preferred method is officially making a comeback) or other contraceptive devices like the ParaGard IUD.

When will the effects of pregnancy go away post-delivery?

Not until the kid hits 18! Ha, I joke. A little.

Now that you are no longer pregnant, you're chomping at the bit to regain your pre-pregnancy body. Trust me, I TOTALLY GET IT! But remember, you didn't acquire all this extra weight and fluid overnight, so you aren't likely to lose it overnight. The good news is you will readily shed at least six to eight pounds at delivery (depending on the weight of the baby), a pound or so due to the weight of the placenta, as well as a few pounds from the weight of all the extra fluid volume you have been toting around to support the pregnancy. That's easily ten to 12 pounds just from the delivery itself! But now for the other side of that coin. Remember when I said swelling usually gets worse post-delivery before it gets better? Well, it's the truth. Now that you are no longer pregnant, your body has to reabsorb, redistribute, and get rid of all the fluids that were necessary to maintain your pregnancy. That, combined with the additional IV fluids you likely received during labor all contribute to you feeling like the abominable snowwoman. My general recommendations as they pertain to swelling are to ingest plenty of fluids. Water with lemon is my personal fave, as well as propping your feet up when you have time. Your kidneys will kick into overdrive and you will have to pee like it's going out of style, but this will kick-start the fluid run-off process. You'll also sweat plenty of the extra fluid off.

While I encourage my pregnant moms to exercise during the course of their pregnancies because of all the benefits it provides, post-delivery is a fine time to initiate healthy eating habits and establish a workout regimen to support you as you get that pre-pregnancy body back. I usually suggest starting with light cardio and progressing as your body sees fit. If you delivered by C-section, I do not recommend any abdominal work until you are at least eight weeks post-delivery and have been cleared by your obstetrician. Now that's a Godsend if I've ever heard one: no core workouts for eight weeks! *Clouds part and angels descend*

As for the rest of the changes your body will undergo post-delivery, now that your hormonal levels of both estrogen and progesterone are rapidly declining, here are a few things you might notice:

Your hair starts shedding: The same way the increase in hormones caused your hair to become voluminous during the pregnancy, we see the opposite effect now that your hormonal levels are dropping. This shedding is most noticeable during the first few months post-delivery but evens out thereafter.

Skin, oh skin: The skin undergoes many changes during the course of the pregnancy. Some women experience stretch marks, darkening in certain areas, acne, or perhaps improved skin aka that pregnancy glow. Post-delivery, with the drop in hormonal levels, stretch marks and those dark spots that you noted during the course of your pregnancy (for example, that line down the middle of your belly known as the linea nigra) will lighten. Stretch marks, while they will also fade, may not completely disappear.

I experienced the worst acne in the world during my pregnancy, so much so that I cried! I shouldn't have worried because, post-delivery, my skin cleared up beautifully due primarily to the decrease in hormones as well as witch hazel pads (unsolicited beauty tip for you). Some of you may experience the opposite effect and note that you have worsening acne, again, due to the decrease in hormones post-delivery.

The breast: Your breast milk usually comes in about two to three days post-delivery. This can be characterized by your breasts becoming very full, tender, and downright painful. You may also experience a fever. This is nothing that a little Tylenol or Motrin won't resolve.

The cramping that is associated with breastfeeding is entirely normal. If your labor was induced, then you are probably familiar with the medication Pitocin. Well, when you breastfeed, the brain releases a chemical that differs from Pitocin by only one carbon. That chemical is called oxytocin. Just as Pitocin makes your uterus contract, so does oxytocin. You can decrease the likelihood of breast engorgement, which is characterized by breast fullness, heaviness, hardness, and even a low-grade fever, by feeding as soon after delivery as possible, frequent breastfeeding (as often as 8 to 12 times per day), as well as massaging the feeding breast while the baby is nursing. If you experience continued breast pain, flu-like symptoms, and a fever greater than or equal to 101.5 degrees, your OB/GYN should be contacted, as what may have initially been engorgement may have evolved into mastitis (an infection of the breast).

To breastfeed or not to breastfeed. That is still the question. Remember, breastfeeding is a very personal choice. While I could write a book about the benefits of breastfeeding, ranging from the passive immunity against certain illnesses passed on to baby via breast milk to the decreased risk of infants being affected by certain illnesses (stomach viruses and lower respiratory infections are only two that I'll mention here). I could also write a book equally as lengthy about why women choose not to breastfeed.

I was one of those women who chose not to breastfeed! It seems a bit blasphemous that as an OB/GYN I would choose not to breastfeed, but everyone who knows me, my friends, even my wife, all knew that breastfeeding would not be for me, and they were right. Not breastfeeding was a personal decision. For all those moms who choose to do it, more power to you. To those moms that choose not to: IT'S OKAY! And guess what, my kid, as well as all the other kids who were not breastfed, turned out just fine. I share this not to go on a soapbox or to champion one cause over the other. I only share this to let you know that either way, it's okay. IT'S YOUR CHOICE!

For those of you not breastfeeding, avoiding breast stimulation, wearing a tight bra, and applying cold packs to the breast (and you thought those frozen packs of vegetables just sitting in your freezer would never be good for anything) will help in getting your milk to dry up.

The vagina: The usual recommendation post-delivery is vaginal rest until you have been seen by your OB at your six-week postpartum visit. This is to ensure that the vagina has had an adequate amount of time to heal and recover after the birth of the baby. If by chance you have a laceration that was repaired at the time of delivery, your sutures will dissolve on their own (INSERT HUGE SIGH OF RELIEF HERE) in about six weeks.

Regarding intercourse post-delivery, make sure you use a heavy lubricant! With the declining hormonal levels post-delivery, the vagina is not nearly as lubricated as it usually is, hence it may be a bit dry and therefore intercourse may be painful (to say the least). Also, if you are breastfeeding, this act in and of itself lends itself to producing a low estrogen state in the body, which contributes to less lubrication in the vagina, which can lead to more painful intercourse. In a nutshell, my advice is to use a lubricant with sex post-delivery.

MISCELLANEOUS

When should I call my OB/GYN?

Signs of labor are a very common topic of discussion within the professional obstetric community, especially as a patient gets closer and closer to her due date.

While I encourage all of my patients to call ANYTIME, here are my top five reasons to call your OB:

1. You think your water broke!

STOP THE PRESSES! PUMP THE BRAKES! You need to call your OB immediately! Whether you are full-term or pre-term, this is a really big deal. I am occasionally amazed at patients who casually arrive a day or two after the fact as if nothing has occurred. If your membranes have ruptured (sorry for the scary technical verbiage), you need to be evaluated so that the proper steps can be taken to ensure a good outcome.

In some instances, this may mean moving towards delivery. In other circumstances, it may mean administering antibiotics. Regardless, an evaluation needs to happen expeditiously so that appropriate action can be taken.

2. You are having regular contractions!

Everyone's definition of regular is different. I typically advise my patients as follows:

If you're having contractions, or regular uterine tightening, occurring seven minutes or less apart while more than an hour has transpired and those contractions are still happening with the frequency noted, you need to call your OB immediately! Unfortunately, labor isn't something I can predict over the phone, so as annoying as I know it can be to have to drive all the way to the hospital only to be told it's a false alarm, remember, I too have to come in and evaluate you.

The consequences of not coming in for an evaluation are numerous, to say the least. A few consequences right off the top of my head are not getting appropriate antibiotic treatment if you are group B strep positive, missing the opportunity to get an epidural if you desire one, and, my personal favorite, ending up with a drive-thru delivery. You know what I'm talking about, right, just making it to the front of the hospital, delivering the baby in the car, only to be wheeled up to labor and delivery in a wheelchair for the doctor to deliver the placenta! No milkshake and fries at the pull-up window here though, so get in early.

3. Bleeding!
If you are truly bleeding (more than just spotting when you wipe, or blood tinged mucous) you need to call your OB immediately.

4. My baby is not moving!
You all know my line. "Is baby movin' and groovin'?" I typically encourage my patients to start doing fetal kick counts at around week 28 of pregnancy. If baby isn't meeting criteria (ten discrete movements over a two-hour time span), or if you aren't feeling the baby move at all, please don't wait until the office opens on Monday, or two to three days after the fact to mention this to your physician. You need to call your OB immediately!

5. You're just not sure.
Whether it's questions about what meds you can take for a cold or headache, you think you might be in labor, or if you are leaking fluid, you need to call your OB immediately!

There are NEVER any dumb questions. As previously stated, you cannot always be sure whether the main event has arrived. Losing your mucus plug, unexplained nausea or diarrhea, they all might just be signs of early labor. These clearly aren't as obvious as some of the ones mentioned above. Remember what G.I. Joe says, "Knowing is half the battle!" So, ask away and get the answers you deserve.

How do you know if the baby's head is down?
This is an extremely common question. There are a few ways to tell whether or not the baby is head-down. The most obvious way is to do a quick ultrasound to confirm position. This is usually my last resort as the other methods typically confirm presentation prior to this one. Those other methods would be a cervical exam and Leopold's maneuvers.

Concerning cervical exams, which you will inevitably get at some point during your pregnancy, while your cervix is being checked, your OB can feel the presenting part to determine whether or not there is a head there. If there is ever any doubt, or if there is no presenting part, an ultrasound can be, and is often, done to confirm presentation.

Leopold's maneuvers, which, by most standards, are pretty old-school, is another method of determining fetal presentation. I like to mix the old with the new, you know that. My patients know that I perform these maneuvers pretty regularly because not only do they give me some idea of fetal presentation and lie (is the baby laying up and down inside your uterus or sideways, aka transverse), but they help me estimate fetal weight. So, if you're reading this and thinking to yourself, OH, that's what Dr. Angela is doing when she's feeling on my uterus, shifting gently from side to side and positioning her hands in various arrangements, whether it be on the fundus, above the pubic symphysis, or along the sides of my uterus, let me tell you, yes. EXACTLY! Again, if all else fails, the ultrasound is the fallback as there's no easier way to determine or confirm presentation aside from actually seeing it. What is it that they say, seeing is believing?

If my baby is breech on an ultrasound, does that mean the baby will stay that way?

NO! Firstly, it depends on when the ultrasound was performed. I don't get too worried about baby's position in the uterus until around the 36th week of gestation. Why? Because up until this point, most babies still have an adequate amount of room to flip, turn, and do cartwheels. And while I know this seems to be a bit of an exaggeration, there's a reason why I ask, "Is baby movin' and groovin'?"

When pregnant mamas get to around 36 weeks or so, we will often discuss how the character of baby's movements may change from the aforementioned cartwheels and somersaults to more subtle activities such as rocking and twisting. This change is typically due to baby not having nearly as much space to move around inside the uterus. Now, that's not to say that baby still can't change from a breech presentation to head-down beyond the 36th week of gestation. In patients that we are performing a C-section on for malpresentation, breech for example, we always perform an ultrasound prior to going to surgery as I have seen babies turn at the last minute.

If my baby is born early, will it be okay?

The answer to this question is, I hope so, it just depends on how early. This question makes me think back to my own pregnancy. Being an OB/GYN and all I obviously know a thing or two about pregnancy. Before every prenatal visit, I always held my breath until I heard those fetal heart tones on the Doppler. Even though I/we had felt our lovebug movin' and groovin' all along, there's nothing like the sound of that heartbeat. I didn't completely let out a sigh of relief until we reached 34 weeks gestation. Why 34 weeks gestation? Because this is a huge milestone! Beyond this week's gestation, there is no intervention that we give regarding trying to arrest labor in an effort to administer steroids for fetal lung maturity. I knew that if I went into labor at 34 weeks, in all likelihood, my bundle of joy would have a fighting chance, specifically with the perinatologists (high-risk physicians for expectant mothers), neonatologists (high-risk doctors for newborns), and all the expertise they had and continue to offer.

While no one wants to have a premature infant, keep this in mind: Even at 37 completed weeks you are still considered early term. The change in nomenclature came about as a result of data showing that babies born at 37 weeks gestation didn't always have similar outcomes to those infants born at 39 weeks gestation. Thus, the American College of Obstetricians and Gynecologists (ACOG) strongly discourages elective inductions (inducing labor without a medical indication) prior to 39 weeks gestation. As noted by the studies, even babies born at full-term can end up in the neonatal intensive care unit.

Should I take a birth class/parenting class?

This is entirely up to you!

I recently shared with some labor and delivery nurses that I did not take a birthing class and, of course, their natural response was, "Why do you need to take a birthing class, you're an OB/GYN?" Well, that meant absolutely nothing! I didn't know anything about taking care of a baby or being anyone's mother. I only had a nephew that I saw on holidays. Honestly, I didn't fit the profile of a person that you would consider a good mom! Remember, at the time of delivery I catch the baby and hand him/her off to the mom. That was, prior to having my daughter, the extent of my interaction with children.

I share the above to simply say get in where you fit in. If you are a person who needs something more structured to build your confidence and make you feel more prepared, then take the classes. If you are like me, more of a fly-by-the-seat-of-her-pants kinda gal, someone who knew that she and her wife would be fine because, number one, we weren't the types to panic, and two, we had a plethora of family, friends, and community to rely on for wisdom, input, remedies, and the occasional funny stories to help get us through. If you're like that, then maybe the classes are not for you.

Just make sure that you utilize your OB/GYN to ask any and all questions you might have. Even when my patients decide to enroll in these classes, they inevitably bring back questions for clarification.

In other news, I don't think you can ever truly be prepared for either childbirth or parenting. Even with every resource at your fingertips, it is just something that you have to experience.

How often will I see my OB/GYN?

Generally speaking, every four weeks, or once a month until you reach 28 weeks or so. THEN, you move to seeing your OB/GYN every two weeks, or twice a month. Once you reach 36 weeks, you will see your OB/GYN weekly. NOW, this time template is based on the assumption that your pregnancy is low risk and uncomplicated. Having said that, I always tell my patients, if there is something going on in your pregnancy that warrants closer monitoring, we will see you accordingly.

In some high risk pregnancies, whether it be multiple gestations (twins for example), insulin dependent gestational diabetes, hypertensive disorders, etc., where closer monitoring is warranted, we may see you as often as twice a week for antepartum testing (whether that be ultrasounds to monitor fetal growth, or biophysical profiles/non stress tests to ensure fetal well-being) once you reach a certain gestational age.

What do I need to know about placental location (previa)?

I typically hear/observe a reference to placental location after a 1st trimester screening ultrasound or after a patient has had their second trimester anatomy scan. Typical placental location is either at the top or sides of the uterus. When the placenta covers the cervix either partially or completely, this is referred to as a previa. A previa occurs when the embryo implants into the lower segment of the uterus. If the placenta only partially covers the cervix and this is noted "earlier" in the pregnancy, there is a greater chance that as the uterus expands, the placental location will "migrate" in such a way that it no longer covers the cervix. If the placenta covers the cervix in its entirety and is noted "later" in the pregnancy, there is a larger probability that the previa will persist and may thus prove to be problematic during the pregnancy.

Outside of ultrasound, painless bleeding, is the major presenting sign/symptom of placenta previa. When I was involved with obstetric resident education, I would often warn the residents against ever doing a digital cervical exam on a pregnant woman with bleeding unless they were certain of placental location. You don't want to do a digital exam on a woman with a previa unless your wish is to get into A LOT of bleeding! The issue with previas is that they are an indication for delivery by C-section. If you are currently or have ever been diagnosed with a placenta previa, pelvic rest is a must, and you usually have instructions to "take it easy" and avoid exercise, strenuous activity, or ANYTHING that might increase your chances of bleeding. You may or may not have episodes of bleeding that require transfusion or even admission to the hospital for closer observation. At times, depending on the severity of the bleed, there may be an indication for early delivery or even an emergency C-section for either maternal or fetal indications.

Risk factors for placenta previa include things such as: previous history of placenta previa, a history of surgery on the uterus whether that be a previous C-section or a myomectomy (fibroid removal), advanced maternal age (age greater than 35), or a multiple gestation (e.g., a twin pregnancy).

What happens if I fall while I'm pregnant?

The big deal is concern for placental abruption or more simply put, separation of the placenta from the uterus resulting from the sheering force of the fall. Anytime I have a patient that is status post any type of abdominal trauma, whether it be from a fall, a motor vehicle accident, or, an odd example I know… getting hit in the uterus while officiating a game of kickball, she needs an evaluation and fetal monitoring.

The usual line of questioning includes: is baby moving and grooving? Are you having any contractions? Are you having any vaginal bleeding? At a minimum, you will require 4-6 hours of fetal and uterine monitoring to observe for contractions and potentially ensuing labor, as well as any changes in fetal status. Though abruption is more of a clinical diagnosis; an ultrasound to evaluate both the placenta and fetus may or may not be ordered. If you are Rh negative, you will likely receive a dose of RhoGAM to prevent any sensitization from a potential blood exchange between you and baby, whose blood type to this point is unknown.

Accessory milk glands, what are they?

Okay, so now that I know I'm not the only one who has experienced this, I'll share my story.

So, I'm moving along, as previously mentioned, not so seamlessly through my pregnancy, remember, I have already told you how miserable I was during my pregnancy between the degenerating fibroid which was painful as all get out, to the awful reflux/heartburn that resulted in about 4 cavities post-delivery. Anyone that knows me knows that this killed me as we are real teeth people in my house.

Anyway, I'm in the third trimester, probably around 36 weeks or so and my breasts are as large as they have ever been (YES!!!) when all of a sudden, I notice this lump in my axilla (that's the region in the upper outer quadrant of your breast leading into your armpit).

OMG, I HAVE BREAST CANCER!!!!

I was so afraid! I was like, "what the heck is this?" It was a pretty decent size and tender, THEN, all of a sudden, it came to me, the accessory milk glands/milk line and its NORMAL distribution.

Because it was difficult for me to function as both a patient and physician, I often struggled with feeling "normal" pregnancy things and self-diagnosing. Due to the hormones of pregnancy, it is NOT uncommon for extra breast tissue to become enlarged, or tender at some point during the pregnancy or postpartum period. Typically, this will resolve on its own; if it doesn't, I treat it just like any other breast lesion and proceed with imaging. Whenever I see a patient experiencing this, I smile inside as I recall how freaked out I was when it happened to me.

That first period postpartum, why is it such a beast?

I get asked this question so often that I routinely address it with my patients when discussing what to expect post-delivery. What I commonly hear is, "why didn't anyone tell me that my period was going to be THAT heavy?" Giving me a bit of a heads up surely would've been appreciated."

That first period post-delivery truly is a BEAST! I remember getting my own period after child birth, mine came a bit sooner than most as I didn't breastfeed. There was so much bleeding and clots I felt like an extra in a Friday the 13th movie! While that is a bit of an exaggeration, there was quite a bit of bleeding, clots, tissue, etc.

Not to fear, however, as this is pretty par for the course. Remember, your hormones are still all over the place and you are still dealing with the lochia that is associated with the postpartum period, if you will recall, I mentioned that lochia can last up to 6 weeks post-delivery.

The reason to remind you of lochia, is that it is associated with discharge, sloughing of tissue, etc., all related to the delivery. This, in addition to your period post-delivery, equals a LOT of blood, tissue, etc. So, as a heads up, get ready, and remember, I don't get too alarmed about postpartum bleeding unless you are bleeding more than a pad per hour. If that occurs, call your OB/GYN immediately.

Pregnancy and Pets

Pets are an irreplaceable part of our families and our lives. Hell, let's admit it, some of us treat pets better than we treat other human beings. I know our lab/boxer mix Franklin lives a better life than many folks I know. I mean, he sleeps most of the day, stays at a five-star pet haven when we travel (at this haven he gets groomed, play sessions with his friends, and his favorite treats which typically include Kongs filled with either yogurt or peanut butter), and gets loved up on by all in the house, with the exception of my wife. She and the dog truly do have a love/hate relationship.

I mention my wife, as she is the one who really made it clear to me that we needed to start implementing some behavioral modifications in our pets prior to the birth of our daughter. Prior to Francesca being born, the dogs were jumping all on the furniture, sleeping in our bed, they were just all over the place! When behaviors such as these have been tolerated over an extended period of time, don't just think that when baby comes home they will miraculously cease! Maybe in your dreams! In reality, is it fair for you to expect such a drastic change in your pet/pets overnight?

So, after some very hard convincing, I finally got on board with reprogramming our dogs regarding what would and what would not be tolerated in our home, all in preparation for the arrival of our precious cargo. I mean, I felt bad; who wants to sleep on the floor? Who wants to watch a movie and not lay on the sofa? Then my wife broke it down for me – Angela, they are dogs! They are thrilled just to be in the house!

This was also a good lesson in parenting. You have to learn to be the leader in your home, not friends! While I love my dogs, the fact of the matter was, they needed to not sleep on the bed anymore or jump on us or the furniture because they could hurt the baby! After I said that to myself a few hundred times, it finally sank in that I was doing the right thing, and the side-eyed glances that the dogs occasionally shot me in their efforts to try to get me to let them back on the furniture became less effective.

How we did it. In retrospect, it was pretty easy. We stopped beckoning them to come sit/lay with us on the furniture. When we found them lounging on the sofa or bed we made them get off. I guarantee you it hurt me more than it hurt them. Where have we heard that before?

In preparation for Francesca's arrival, we sent home blankets, hats, anything with her scent on it so that the dogs would know her when she came home. We also recorded her crying and played it for the dogs prior to her coming home. I found that these things helped a lot.

We NEVER left Francesca alone in a room with the dogs. We also made sure that we showered the dogs with extra love, treats, and attention. After all, this is/was a huge adjustment for them as well. One of the things we found was that the dogs seemed to intuitively know just how special our love bug was. Their allegiance seemed to shift from being our dogs, to being her dog. We soon realized that our focus needed to shift from worrying about the dogs hurting the baby to showing our love bug how to interact with the dogs - no rough treatment, no ear or tail pulling and no riding them like ponies.

For those of you with cats, same rules apply.

You've probably been warned about changing cat litter and the risks of Toxoplasmosis. Well here's the deal with Toxoplasmosis. The reality is that most of us have already been exposed to it. We can check for this by screening your blood for antibodies. Toxoplasmosis is a protozoa that can be contracted either via direct contact or inhalation. Here are a few recommendations for you cat lovers:

Try to avoid changing the cat litter. If there is no way around this, wear gloves.

Change the cat litter daily; little known fact, it takes one to five days for the toxoplasma to become infectious once shed in cat poop.

Keep your cat indoors as much as possible. This avoids contact with other cats/strays that might be infected. Remember, your cat is a predator. They like to hunt. Keeping your cat indoors avoids exposure to mice, birds, or other rodents that might be carriers.

URBAN MYTHS
PREGNANCY OLD WIVES TALES

Are those old wives' tales of pregnancy true?

I LOVE THIS QUESTION!

I cannot begin to tell you how many hee-larious stories I hear about something expectant moms have been told by friends or family predicting things about their unborn child. Determining the sex of the baby or whether or not baby will be born with lots of hair are just a couple of the most common.

As most of the prenatal visits are spent talking about the pregnancy, there is always time for general chit-chat. These pregnancy old wives' tales always seem to be a source of, not only education, as I have found differences in the nature of the wives' tales based on both the age and cultural background of the moms-to-be, but also a source of enormous entertainment!

These old wives' tales come up so often, whether it's one of my patients making a casual remark such as, "The heartbeat is fast, does that mean we're having a girl?" or "I'm having terrible heartburn, that must mean baby has a lot of hair, right?" that I HAD to investigate just a bit more.

Being the scientific mind that I am, I'm still waiting on the data to prove or disprove these sayings, but in the meantime, I decided to interview scores of folks ranging from my more senior patients to expectant moms in search of more understanding and hilarity. This served not only as a learning experience, but yet another opportunity to get to know you, my amazing patients.

While I received scores of feedback, these tales ranged from jaw-droppingly weird to blatantly offensive to downright, fall-over-laughing ridiculous. I decided to narrow down the list to the top ten tales I think you'll enjoy the most. Please know that these are merely old wives' tales and are meant purely for your enjoyment!

AMUSING PREGNANCY MYTHS

1. Girls steal their mother's beauty, boys enhance their mother's beauty.
2. If you experience a lot of heartburn during your pregnancy, your baby will be born with a lot of hair.
3. When asked to show her hands, if a pregnant woman shows her palms up she is having a girl, if she shows her palms down she is having a boy.
4. If there's a food you like or crave a lot during pregnancy, the baby will have a birthmark resembling the shape of that food.
5. If your urine is bright yellow, you're having a boy, if it's dull in color, you're having a girl.
6. You will deliver three days before or after nine full moons.
7. If you are upset with someone during your pregnancy, the child will be born resembling that person.
8. If you crave meat and cheese during your pregnancy, you're having a boy.
9. If you raise your hands over your head while pregnant, the umbilical cord will be wrapped around the baby's neck.
10. If you're carrying high you are having a girl; if you are carrying low you are having a boy.

Bonus for the one I hear ALL the time:
If the fetal heart rate is high, you're having a girl; if the fetal heart rate is low, you're having a boy.

WHERE MY DADS AT?

Remember that 90's jam by the group 702, Where My Girls At? Good single! Really though, where are my dad's at? I pose this question as I can count on one hand the number of fathers-to- be, husbands, boyfriends, baby daddies that I see at the prenatal visits. What's up with that? I mean, it's not as if my pregnant moms got that way by themselves.

I often wonder why more fathers-to-be aren't present for prenatal visits. Is it that the preggo moms don't want them present? If so, I would totally get it! I mean, how often (especially if you have other children) do you have a moment to just get away, even if it is only to your appointment? On the flip side, perhaps there is a conflict in schedules that doesn't allow the significant other to be present at the prenatal visits. I'm all about giving folks the benefit of the doubt, perhaps fathers-to-be don't think that any of what is/will be discussed is applicable to them, even though the last time I checked, this was your baby as well. Maybe you, fathers-to-be, are so overwhelmed, nervous, and/or scared, that you are afraid to come. Whatever the reason, I strongly encourage you to come to as many visits as possible. During my pregnancy my wife came to every visit. She even scheduled visits that I didn't need. This may have had something to do with the fact that I was not the most compliant patient in the world. Had it not been for my wife, I would not have taken my prenatal vitamins, had my lab work done (I'm terribly afraid of needles) and done all the other things that a mother-to-be should do. I was sort of what you would call a royal pain! My prenatal visits were truly more for my wife than myself, as most of the time at these visits my colleague and I discussed office business, other patients, and other things having to do with the practice. Remember, my colleague served not only as my obstetrician, but she was also a dear friend. We had to make an effort to go over all those things that routinely occur at a prenatal visit as a means of helping my wife feel more connected with the pregnancy; otherwise, my visits would've gone pretty much like this…

My OB: "Ang, how are you?"

Me: "Just swell."

My OB: "Is there anything we need to discuss?" (Remember, as an OB, I had a working knowledge of lab results, etc.).

Me: "Not really," and we would move on.

Just as my wife attended every prenatal visit to feel connected, I encourage you, the father-to-be to attend the visits to feel connected. Not only will you see first-hand everything that your wife is going through, but you will also see how far along baby is, what's happened so far, and what to expect in the future. Also, you can get answers to burning questions like (as one of my expectant dads once posed to me), "Dr. Angela, is my wife's vagina supposed to be that big?"

Needless to say, we all had a HUGE laugh! For the record dads, big vaginas, leaking/enlarged breasts, swollen hands and fingers (I've seen pregnant moms wearing their wedding ring sets on their pinky fingers like The Last Don) are all completely normal and par for the course. You learn a lot at the prenatal visits.

So just what is your wife/baby momma going through? For most of you, you experienced five minutes (okay, I'll give you the benefit of the doubt, seven minutes of pleasure to have made this pregnancy possible). Now the expectant mom is left to endure all of the associated pains of pregnancy. Can we say nausea and vomiting? What about pelvic pressure, gas like you wouldn't believe, hemorrhoids? Not to mention having to go to the bathroom like ALL THE TIME, and the discharge that just won't stop? How about heartburn, back pain, swollen feet and ankles? I'm sure I'm leaving out scores of other symptoms that pregnant moms experience on a routine basis.

Another obvious reason I love when significant others show up at prenatal visits is that you serve as my second set of eyes and ears. Pregnancy brain can greatly affect an expectant mom's memory, so it's nice to have fathers/partners/wives around to fill in the blanks. Those questions that mom can't remember, often you do. You also serve as a good means of ensuring that expectant mothers are being compliant with recommended treatment, whether it is following a specific diet or not overdoing it with activities.

You are a constant source of motivation, encouragement, and strength. Pregnancy is difficult enough as it is. Knowing that you are there every step of the way is PRICELESS! All the "little" things like showering your expectant mom with compliments of how beautiful she is, rubbing her feet, painting her toes, and giving back rubs/massages go a very long way. I guarantee you that most moms do not feel beautiful during the course of pregnancy. We/they feel like, and this is a direct quote, WHALES. Remember I shared the story of myself crying inside my walk-in closet at around six weeks because I could no longer fit into any of my clothes. While my wife later confided in me that it took everything in her not to burst out laughing at such utter ridiculousness, her coming in, sitting on the floor reassuring me that I was still thebomb.com, and as beautiful as ever, and that we would find a fantastic wardrobe that fit, made me feel like a million bucks. I have never, and will never, forget that.

Dads, coming to prenatal visits is a way to let expectant moms know that they aren't in this alone. It also gives you a better understanding of all the changes that are occurring in the mom-to-be. And you thought she was just making all of this up! What does GI Joe say? *"Knowing is half the battle?"* Now you will have a better understanding of why your partner is moody, irritable, and craving everything under the sun. Not to mention, coming to the prenatal visits will give you some clue as to how far along your wife/partner/baby's mama actually is. If you come regularly to the prenatal visits you'll know what signs and symptoms of labor to keep your eyes peeled for so that if in fact you are the one calling me at some God-awful hour in the morning, you have some idea of what is going on and can speak on our pregnant patient's behalf if necessary. I tell you, there is nothing worse than getting a call from a significant other who knows absolutely nothing about how far along in the pregnancy the expectant mom is, whether or not her water has broken, and if/how often contractions are occurring. The prenatal visits are your opportunity to get a clue, as well as learn what to anticipate during the actual labor and delivery process.

FROM ONE MOM TO ANOTHER

I absolutely loved writing this book. It is a constant reminder of why I do what I do. Pregnant women are the best!

Pregnancy is exciting. Nerve wracking. Scary. Unpredictable.

Once upon a time I had no idea what pregnancy was really all about. I mean, from a textbook and clinical perspective, yes, but experiencing it is a whole different thing. My own pregnancy journey enabled me to be a better physician by allowing me to relate, and better understand, just what my pregnant moms were experiencing when they dished on crazy cravings or debilitating back pain or the endless urge to pee. No longer could I roll my eyes, in my mind, of course, or dismiss my patients' nonstop complaining about swollen feet or not feeling sexy anymore. Finally, I really got it, and to all the expectant mamas out there, I still completely get it.

My hope is that this book will serve as a guide to support you through your own pregnancy. Through my own personal stories, shared experiences, and belief in a simple, old-school approach to life, let this work be a reminder that you are not alone. You are not the only one who feels all these wild emotions or has experienced these outrageous bodily changes. I hope this book serves as a reminder that you are beautiful, and that it's all worth it.

Remember, nobody is born knowing how to be a mom. As long as you do the best that you can it will be good enough, for you and your brand-new bouncing baby.

Until next time,

Look Better. Feel Better. Be Better.

Dr. Angela.

ABOUT THE AUTHOR

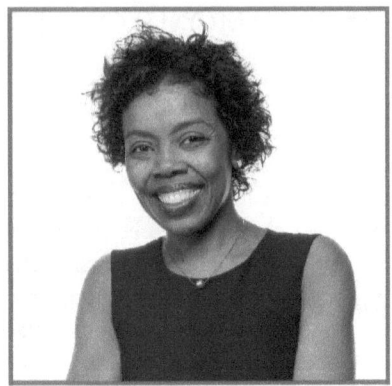

Wife, mother, Midwesterner, and award-winning OB/GYN, Dr. Angela is equal parts best girlfriend and bold professional, supporting women's health with innovative approaches to care and heavy doses of humor. Dr. Angela has done more than launch a successful practice, she has defined herself as a voice for a new generation of womanhood, established her *ASK DR. ANGELA* brand committed to authenticity, and built a community rooted in trust, candor, and compassion.

www.ingramcontent.com/pod-product-compliance
Lightning Source LLC
Chambersburg PA
CBHW031235280526
45784CB00004B/1580